THE PALEO

Easy Recipes

Author

Ellen J. Burns

Contents

Budgeting Key #1: Avoid making dishes that center around premium products. I like to get the most bang for my buck. To do this, I avoid making dishes that center around premium products. Even something like bacon can really run up your grocery bill if it becomes a staple ingredient on the weekly meal rotation or is treated as a main protein like chicken or beef. I also rarely make Paleo treats, which so often call for larger quantities of pricey items like nuts and nut flours, pure maple syrup, raw honey and so on. It's not that I don't purchase and cook with those ingredients, only that I typically avoid recipes that call for large quantities of them.

Many recipes in this book call for ingredients that aren't inherently budget-friendly choices, but you will notice that the ingredient is used sparingly. So have bacon; just don't eat it for breakfast every day. Drizzle on some raw honey or pure organic maple syrup; just avoid preparing recipes that require a lot of it. You'll spend $20 every few months versus every few weeks when you avoid making dishes that center around premium products.

Budgeting Key #2: Think simple. Let's face it, it's easy to get distracted by food porn. You know, those impressive recipes with exotic ingredients, nearly all of which replicate non-Paleo junk food favorites or indulgences. They can make us feel like we're doing it wrong if we enjoy a simple baked sweet potato, steamed broccoli, a few organic raspberries and some grilled chicken. Truth is, the actual daily Paleo life looks way more like the latter than the former. Don't get suckered into thinking that you need to make this harder than you really do.

Think about it this way. Scrap the idea of Paleo for a second and consider making dinner for yourself on an average Thursday night. Does your mind leap to gourmet ingredients and intricate culinary methods? My guess is likely not. Before I was Paleo, a typical weeknight dinner would generally be centered around a starch (quick to prepare and filling), and then I'd determine a protein partner based on which item in the meat drawer demanded eating first. Lastly, I'd come up with a quick sauce and maybe a vegetable side. That was dinner. Never in a million years would you catch me making pasta from scratch or making a trip to a specialty market to pick up a $15 spice on a random weeknight.

My point? Most meals are a matter of meeting our need for food as conveniently as possible and with minimal effort. So why complicate that when it comes to the Paleo diet? Purchasing quality ingredients with the intention of approachable preparations is one of the best ways to maximize your grocery budget. Keep it simple.

Budgeting Key #3: Pick a side. Fact is, it's very difficult to live a double-diet life and not expect to spend twice the money on food. Purchasing both premium, nutrient-dense whole foods for primary meal sources in addition to refined, processed faux-foods for snacks and lazy meals, which cost a great deal in relation to their nutritive qualities, is a money burner for sure. In fact, let me share a story with you on this.

My husband often travels for work, and one time early in our Paleo journey I decided to experiment with our budget during his absence. I wanted to see how preparing only Paleo meals and snacks for four would affect our monthly food costs. The kids even followed suit, though most of the time they didn't realize they were Paleo, too, thanks to homemade gummy snacks made with grass-fed gelatin; green smoothies loaded with berries, spinach and avocado; and, of course, plantain and coconut chips made with coconut oil and sprinkled with cinnamon. Would you believe it if I told you that in one month I was able to reduce our food spending by $1,000? I was floored, too. And actually, so was my husband. After this experiment, we knew we were on to something.

I did it by making some very simple and straightforward adjustments that anyone can do. The first was cutting out routine stops at our local coffee shop. Other than an Americano with a splash of cream, some hot tea or good ol' fashioned *temptation*, there really isn't much for us there. Truth be told, I'd rather whip up a quick butter coffee at home anyway.

Next, we ate out much, much less. Our family loves to go out to breakfast on Saturday mornings, then we swing by a coffee shop for a hot cup of something before we go run it off at a park. With dad gone, we skipped the first two steps of that tradition and replaced it with a quick breakfast at home. My kids never turn down special breakfasts with bacon, since it's still considered a treat in our house and not a primary protein source.

The last thing we did which really drove it home for me was that we ate everything I bought at the store. Nothing went to waste. I planned meals and snacks, made them and ate them. It really is that simple. I didn't get suckered into sales or spontaneous buys because I thought something looked or sounded good in that moment. I made a plan and followed through with it. This, of course, was adopted after learning the hard way that I was buying a lot more than I needed.

One time I dropped by the grocery store with the intention of picking up a few items needed for dinner. I walked in with a short list, grabbed a cart and ran through the store quickly. When I was unloading my groceries, I laughed at how many things there were in the bags that were not on my list! After that day I decided that if I only had a few things to pick up, I would grab a hand basket instead of a cart (a habit from corralling kids), and limit the amount of empty space that seemed to whisper, "Fill me up, there's plenty of room."

These simple steps contributed to saving nearly $1,000 in food costs. Amazing, right?

This brings me to my last tip when picking a side: Don't spend your time trying to re-create all your favorite Standard American Diet (SAD) foods with Paleo ingredients! You'll go broke in the process and burn out, and ultimately it'll never taste the same and lead to disappointment, which increases the risk of you walking away altogether. Allow your taste buds for treats, breaded meats or sugary glazes, to evolve alongside the changes occurring on your plate. One day a bowl of fresh berries with a dollop of refined-sugar-free whipped coconut milk may just become the perfect dessert.

Budgeting Key #4: Be Informed. The first thing you'll hear when learning about the Paleo diet is to buy only organic, non-GMO, locally sourced and pasture-raised protein and produce. But what does all that even mean?

Organic food means that the food has been grown and processed without the presence of synthetic fertilizers or pesticides. However, pesticides from natural sources may be used in producing organic food.

What organic does *not* mean is that the food hasn't been genetically modified. Just because something wasn't processed with pesticides doesn't guarantee that it hasn't been genetically engineered. That's a separate check. GMO produce has been intentionally altered so that its DNA contains one or more genes not normally found in its original makeup. In other words, it's

Franken-food. Consumers want their food to last longer, be prettier, taste better and, in general, be larger in size. And there are scientists standing by who are happy to oblige. We don't like apples that go bad after a few days, so someone wearing a lab coat comes along to fix that.

Unfortunately, consuming foods that have been genetically modified has the ability to impact our bodies negatively. After all, if it's not a naturally occurring organism, our bodies often have difficulties knowing how to process the foreigners. Yep, you heard right. Our bodies are xenophobes; they don't like strangers. And when it comes to food, you don't get much stranger than genetically engineered produce and the synthetic chemicals that cultivate and preserve them.

The best quality you can purchase is locally grown, seasonal, organic, non-GMO. However, that's not always realistic. Again, with all things, always keep in mind that it is essential to do your own research and draw conclusions that resonate with you. Be informed about the terms that are thrown around to describe the food you consume and make intentional, realistic decisions for yourself and your family.

For example, were you aware that there are several fruits and vegetables that don't really need to be organic?

The Environmental Working Group (http://www.ewg.org/foodnews) prepared a list of the best and worst fruits and vegetables when it comes to the presence of pesticides to inform consumers which produce really should be organic and which may not pose too great a risk if conventionally grown.

According to the EWG, the fruits and vegetables that retain the most amount of pesticides and chemicals are (listed in order, with apples being the most contaminated):

• Apples

• Strawberries

• Grapes

• Celery

• Peaches

• Spinach

• Sweet bell peppers

• Imported nectarines

• Cucumbers

• Cherry tomatoes

• Imported snap peas

• Potatoes

• Hot peppers

- Domestic blueberries

- Lettuce

Those lowest in pesticides are (listed in order, with avocados being the least contaminated):

- Avocados

- Sweet corn

- Pineapples

- Cabbage

- Frozen sweet peas

- Onions

- Asparagus

- Mangoes

- Papayas

- Kiwifruit

- Eggplant

- Grapefruit

- Cantaloupe

- Cauliflower

- Sweet potatoes

In terms of meat and egg sources, local pasture-raised is always the best. Industrialized meat production has stooped to new lows in the last century. From the way animals are treated to the nutrients their meat yields, it's a negative situation all around. Many people, particularly those in the Paleo community, seek to support local farmers who raise cows, pigs, sheep and chickens in the most ethical and natural manner available. Fresh air, sunshine, rain, mud, insects, grass— these are all elements vital to the life and diet of an ethically raised animal. Withhold or substitute these things, and not only is the handling of the animal compromised, but also the nutritive quality of their meat.

Since many of us haven't given a second thought to procuring our protein from anywhere other than the local grocery store or wholesale retailer, the concept of buying directly from the producers may be downright strange. Now I'm hoping that's a "strange-cool" instead of "strange-weird" because there are a lot of hardworking people out there who depend on folks like us to take a risk and break away from the norm.

The website www.eatwild.com can help you find local farms where you can buy all of your meat, vegetables, fruits and sometimes even nuts. I used this website to locate one near me, which offers cuts of pastured pigs frozen and ready for immediate sale as well as the opportunity to purchase a hog (in whole or in part) each year. They also host a Community Supported Agriculture (CSA) program where they grow and provide organic vegetables to members each week. I encourage you to spend some time on that website and discover your local resources. Be a little rebellious and buy your food differently.

A FEW THINGS BEFORE YOU GET STARTED COOKING …

Remember that frugal Paleo cooking goes beyond saving money. Your time has value. Your health has value. Your sanity has value.

Value Your Time

Plan your meals each week. But instead of buying into the sales pitch that each night has to jump from gourmet swordfish to elegant duck breast, get cozy with the idea of grilled chicken with a side of sautéed vegetables. Use fresh herbs, a variety of dried spices and some citrus to give your dishes distinction. Meals do not need to be complicated!

Here's a tip for meal planning that has been a proven winner for me: Pick a flavor profile each week and shop accordingly. Sticking with a food theme for the week helps to narrow the scope of ingredients you shop for, which results in savings. So as an example, for a Mexican food themed week, buy lots of avocados, fresh tomatoes, cilantro, pork shoulder for carnitas, beef chuck roast for barbacoa, fresh heads of lettuce for wraps, cauliflower for ricing and a few limes to give your dishes a fresh citrus finish. All of the items you purchase for one recipe are easily rolled forward into another, wasting very little if any of the ingredients purchased.

The bonus of saving time by planning your meals is that you no longer have to worry about what to make in the 11th hour of the day. You've organized your week; you know you have the right ingredients on hand; and you know that you'll be covered for the next day as well.

Cook smart. There are three keys to smart cooking. The first is to familiarize yourself with the recipe. Read it over two or three times before you slice your first vegetable. Know this recipe well enough that as you cook, it becomes second nature—or close enough to it.

The second key is to take the time to cut, slice, mince, chop and trim all of the ingredients first before you begin to cook. Prepare and set out everything that will be used in the recipe so that as you progress through it, the ingredients are waiting for you and not the other way around. This allows you to move through the recipe with ease.

The third is to have quality kitchen gear. Use a cast-iron skillet or ceramic glazed Dutch oven. Be sure your knives are sharp. Invest in a good-quality roasting pan and other kitchen equipment as needed. I find that I enjoy cooking a lot more when I have the right tools. Fumbling around with dull knives, thin-bottomed pans that have hot spots and don't evenly cook food, or poor-quality bakeware that causes everything to stick really frustrates me in the kitchen. It makes me not want to cook. Over the years I have found great deals at yard sales and the clearance section at home stores, and I've asked for gift cards to stores that sell quality kitchen items in order to build up equipment that makes cooking fun and convenient.

Remember that scratch is good, but not always best. There are a handful of things that I really don't mind spending the money on versus spending the time on them. It's fairly easy to find a recipe for nearly anything that is typically a processed item. But some of those recipes can be really involved, time consuming or expensive. If it's not feasible to spend hours on a recipe and you are able to access a premade equivalent, by all means, buy it! For example, I'll gladly drop $5 on a bag of sweet potato chips made with coconut oil and sea salt so that I can whip up a batch of Irish Nachos for a Sunday football game without spending the time on chip preparation. For me, it's worth the time savings. However, when it comes to plantain chips, I really like making those myself. I find the texture is better and so is the cost. Ultimately it is a matter of preference, and I encourage you to take the time to assess what is best for your family's lifestyle and budget.

Another point to consider is how far premade foods have come. Word is getting out about the negative effects of gluten, the dangers of soy and the unintended consequences of refined sugars. More and more consumers are calling for healthy alternatives! The good news that comes with this initiative is that folks who share the same passion as you and I are producing amazing Paleo-friendly products like coconut-oil-based dessert items, grain-free pastas, snack bars from dates and nuts, various flavors of kale chips with only natural ingredients and so on. Suddenly we don't *have* to make everything ourselves to ensure we're getting only the best of what nature has to offer. If it is within your means to save some time and purchase an item that maintains Paleo standards premade, then do it.

Value Your Health

It cannot be said enough that Paleo is not a rigid diet fad meant for quick weight loss or anything along those lines. Paleo is a lifestyle which seeks to support individualized optimal health through focused nutrition. It eliminates foods that are known for carrying dietary baggage.

It is important to convey, too, that Paleo is not looking to reenact history or resurrect the exact eating habits of our ancestors, but rather reshape our understanding of what food truly is and how to best nourish these bodies of ours. It's a marriage between ancestral dietary practices and modern analysis. This results in the best of both time periods—pre-industrialized foods scrutinized by advanced science.

Just as dietary needs vary from person to person, so will the practice of Paleo. For example, an athlete's version of Paleo will look drastically different from someone who has adopted the diet for weight loss. Likewise, a person with an autoimmune condition, or who is managing chronic illness with a specific protocol, will eat much differently than a healthy person who is a whole foods lover.

Value your health, identify what your body needs (and does not need) to thrive and eat in a way that best supports it.

Value Your Sanity

Sometimes this Paleo thing is perceived to be too overwhelming to manage as a lifestyle. But many of us who have been practicing for a while will tell you that the opposite is true. It took some practice to get here, though. The key? Instead of focusing on the things you've eliminated, hone in on the foods you want to eat that make you feel great—and give yourself a break from time to time.

Remember that this is not a pass-fail diet. Paleo is highly adaptive and will look different from person to person and family to family. In my family, we are not militant. Unless you have a serious allergy or medical reason to absolutely eliminate a particular ingredient, relax a little bit and make a compromise. In fact, I will tell you that I don't spend a lot of time preparing Paleo desserts. We treat treats as treats in my home, and therefore they do not happen regularly. So when it's time for us to indulge a little, we walk to our neighborhood frozen yogurt joint or doughnut shop and dive right in headfirst! We know that we'll get a headache or a tummy ache and have an energy crash—and our kids will go bonkers for a few hours—and we are fine with that on occasion.

The concept here is that stress can be as harmful as the foods we seek to eliminate, so if you are robbing Peter to pay Paul when it comes to stressing over food, then you've really done little to advance the proverbial ball. Again, if there isn't a serious medical reason not to, save your sanity, save your time, save the money … eat the doughnut.

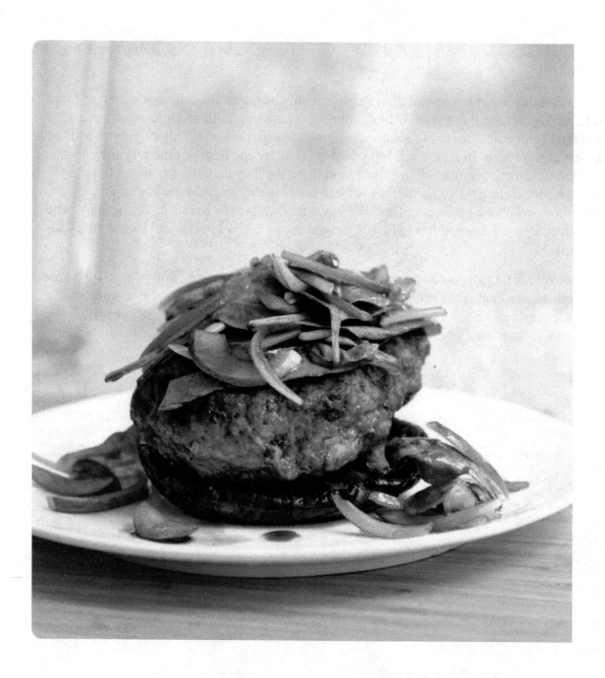

There is such an opportunity to save money with beef! Sure there's tenderloin, filet mignon or a monster porterhouse to nosh on, but they come with premium price tags no matter which way you slice it. We're going to wander away from the budget-breakers and find some shanks and shoulders!

Before we hit the grocery store, remember that quality matters. There's a big nutritive difference between cows that eat soy- and grain-based feed and cows that are pastured, eating lots of grass and soaking up sunshine. When animals eat and live the way they were meant to, we all reap the benefits. In order for us to get critical vitamins, minerals and essential acids from beef, those cows have got to eat grass. Grain- and soy-based feeds do little to nourish cattle, rendering their meat near vacant of important nutrients like omega-3 fatty acids, conjugated linoleic acid (CLA), B and E vitamins, iron and zinc. Consider the cost of purchasing all of those supplements separately. Why not eat grass-fed beef and save yourself the trip to the supplement store? Maximize your meat; eat pastured.

Now let's talk about driving your dinner home with a flavor punch! The best ways to draw out flavor from budget-friendly cuts are roasting, grilling and, in particular, braising. Braising and affordable cuts of meat are a match made in culinary heaven. The low and slow cooking process relaxes those tight connective tissues and lets juices flow, giving you incredible depth of flavor and juicy, tender meat. And that, my friends, is never a bad thing.

And while we're on the subject of getting the best bang for our buck, lest we not forget the hidden jewels of our bovine friends: offal and marrow. Stay with me now. You may not be ready to take such a big leap in your Tuesday night cuisine, but I have a couple of recipes that might nudge you a little closer to the edge. Not only are these cuts easy on the wallet, they are incredibly nourishing! Did you know that gram for gram, beef liver from pastured cows contains more than 18 times the folate found in an apple? Somebody grab me an onion!

It's time to make the most of our beef.

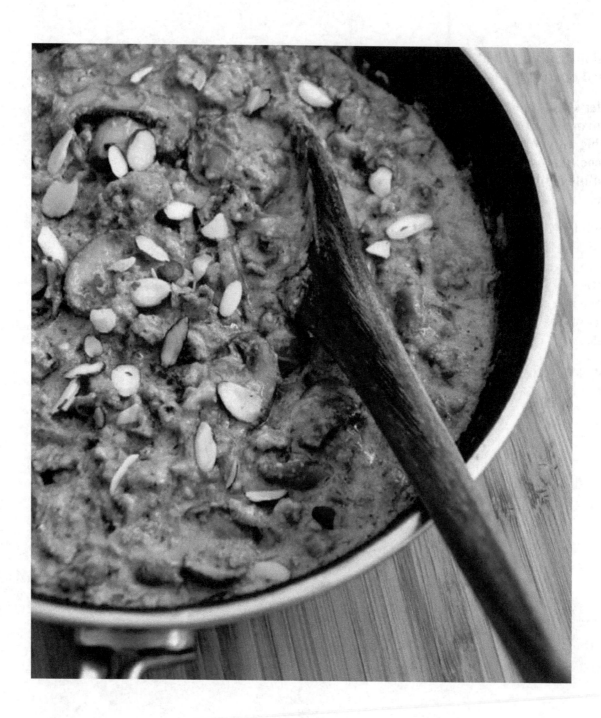

BEEF STROGANOFF

One of the freedoms that comes with the Paleo diet is breaking away from the notion that meaty sauces must be paired with a starch to form a complete dish. That being said, I love to eat this Beef Stroganoff with crunchy kelp noodles, though it is equally fantastic with spaghetti squash. I'm also just as satisfied warming this up for breakfast the next day with a fried over-easy egg on top. If you're a fan of batch cooking for saving time and money, be sure to put this recipe on the rotation!

Serves 6 to 8

2 tbsp (30 g) lard or preferred Paleo-friendly fat

1 large (about 4 inches [10 cm]) white or yellow onion, diced

2 to 3 cloves garlic, minced

3 cups (225 g) white mushrooms, sliced

2 lb (908 g) grass-fed ground beef

1 tsp (5 g) dried oregano

1 tsp (5 g) dried thyme

1 tsp (5 g) coarse sea salt

Black pepper, to taste

2 tbsp (30 mL) apple cider vinegar

2 tbsp (30 mL) arrowroot flour

2 cups (474 mL) almond milk

Sliced almonds, for garnish (optional)

Building the stroganoff will be done in layers starting with the big flavor players: onion and garlic. I prefer to use a Dutch oven for this recipe, but any large high-sided skillet or heavy-bottomed pan will do. Heat it up to medium-high and melt a couple of tablespoons (about 30 to 45 mL) of lard or your preferred Paleo-friendly fat, such as tallow, duck fat, or coconut, olive or avocado oil. Bacon grease would not be wrong here.

Add the onion, garlic and mushrooms first. Cook and stir until the onion is translucent, the garlic fragrant and the mushrooms lightly caramelized, about 7 to 9 minutes. Remove from the pan and set aside.

In the same pan over medium-high heat, replenish the fat if it has dried out any and drop in the beef along with the dry seasonings (oregano, thyme, sea salt and black pepper) and the apple cider vinegar. Cook until the beef has browned. Depending on the amount of moisture in the beef, there may or may not be juice in the pan rendered from the beef once it has cooked through. If there is an excess, do not drain! Move to the next step and consider the extra juices as a flavor bonus for the sauce.

When nearly done, dust the beef with the arrowroot flour. Be sure to mix well so the arrowroot doesn't sit in any pools of rendered fat and juices. Arrowroot is a tricky ingredient and will gel with liquid. We want that thickening to happen in this next step.

Return the onion, garlic and mushrooms to the pan and mix with the beef. Then slowly pour in the almond milk. That arrowroot flour will start to thicken the sauce now. Simmer on medium-low heat, uncovered, until the sauce reaches desired thickness, usually just another 5 to 10 minutes.

Transfer to a large serving bowl or spoon on top of your choice of vegetable or Paleo-friendly noodles in individual serving bowls. Garnish with some sliced almonds on top if you like, but consider it optional since sliced almonds are not always affordable.

SPAGHETTI AND MEATBALL STEW

Say what?! Yep, spaghetti and meatballs ... made into stew. It's one way this Italian mama gets to enjoy a favorite childhood meal. This is hearty, loaded with vegetables and brimming with nourishing bone broth. It's everything I want in a meal. Another perk to this recipe? It makes excellent leftovers for lunch the next day. Cook once, eat at least twice. #winning

Serves 6

FOR THE MEATBALLS

1 lb (454 g) grass-fed ground beef

12 to 16 oz (340 to 454 g) pastured ground pork

½ tsp kosher salt

½ tsp garlic powder

1 egg

FOR THE SOUP

3 tbsp (45 mL) extra virgin olive oil

1 ½ cups (225 g) diced yellow onions

4 cloves garlic, minced

1 cup (150 g) diced carrots

2 cups (450 g) chopped kale

1 tsp (5 g) dried basil

½ tsp sea salt

⅛ tsp ground cinnamon

Pinch of red-pepper flakes

1 (28 oz [794 g]) can organic crushed tomatoes

1 (14.5 oz [411 g]) can organic diced tomatoes

3 cups (711 mL) beef bone broth, homemade preferred

1 (14.5 oz [411 g]) can organic cut green beans

3 small zucchini

Fresh basil or flat-leaf Italian parsley, for garnish (optional)

Let's start with the meatballs. Mix all of the listed ingredients together by hand and roll into equal-size meatballs. You should get 12.

Prepare the vegetables as described and open up the cans, setting everything aside, ready for the soup.

Break out your Dutch oven or large, heavy-bottomed stockpot and heat to medium-high. Add the olive oil to get the pan started. Arrange 4 to 6 meatballs in the pan and begin to brown them. Be sure not to overcrowd the pan or the meatballs will cause the temperature to decrease, resulting in soggy, steaming meatballs and not the crisp, brown crust we need.

Brown the meatballs on at least 2 sides—the centers should be raw; we just want to create a crust. This should take about 3 to 4 minutes per side. Set the browned meatballs aside for later. Repeat until all of the meatballs are browned.

Add a little more olive oil if the pan looks dry. Then toss in the onions, garlic, carrots, kale and dry seasonings (the basil, sea salt, cinnamon and red-pepper flakes). If you're not used to building sauces this way, it may appear a bit strange. This method releases the oils in the dried seasonings, yielding a more flavorful sauce.

When the carrots and kale have softened and the onions become translucent, add the meatballs back to the pot and cover with the canned crushed and diced tomatoes, beef broth and drained green beans. Stir gently and bring to a boil. After the stew bubbles for about 3 to 4 minutes, reduce the temperature to a simmer. Cover and let this stew bubble away for about 30 minutes. Stir just a couple of times during that 30 minutes.

While the stew finishes, grab those zucchini. Trim the ends off and divide them into thirds or about 2-inch sections. Using a spiral slicer or another tool for making quick julienne vegetables, run these zucchini through to make short "noodles."

Place about a cup or so (150 g) of raw zoodles (zucchini + noodle = **zoodles**) in the serving bowls, then ladle in 1 or 2 meatballs and some spaghetti stew. Zoodles overcook easily, so I find that adding them raw directly to the bowl (rather than to the pot) keeps them crisp and their texture more like pasta.

Top with fresh basil or parsley, if you like.

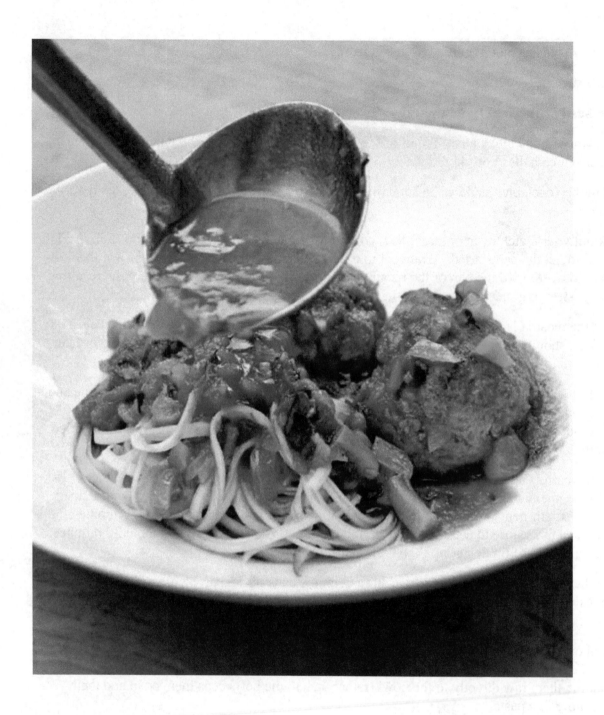

SLOW COOKER ITALIAN BEEF

Some days are just meant for slow cookers. We all have them. So when that day comes, toss this easy beef recipe into the slow cooker, set your timer and tackle the demands of the day with the comfort of knowing you will have a delicious meal awaiting you when it has all been accomplished.

Serves 6

2 ½ to 3 lb (1.1 to 1.4 kg) beef chuck roast

2 cups (400 g) chopped carrots

1 small white or yellow onion, sliced

4 to 5 cloves garlic, chopped

1 tsp (5 g) kosher salt

1 tsp (3 g) garlic powder

1 tsp (3 g) dried basil

1 tsp (3 g) dried oregano

½ tsp dried thyme

⅛ tsp ground cinnamon

Pinch of red-pepper flakes

1 cup (237 mL) organic crushed tomatoes

1 cup (237 mL) homemade beef stock (here)

1 tbsp (13 g) tomato paste

Prepare the beef by trimming off excess fat and cutting the roast into 3- to 4-inch (7.5 to 10 cm) chunks. Place the beef into the slow cooker and move on to the vegetables.

Toss the prepared carrots, onion and garlic in the slow cooker with the beef. Then add the seasonings: kosher salt, garlic powder, basil, oregano, thyme, cinnamon and red-pepper flakes.

Pour in the tomatoes and beef stock. Add the tomato paste and give everything a good stir.

Cover the slow cooker, set to low and cook for 5 to 6 hours. Serve the beef over roasted spaghetti squash with a side of green beans for a low-maintenance meal.

ULTIMATE TACO MEAT

As a mom, when it comes to dinnertime, my first goal is to get my kids to eat as many veggies as possible. My second goal is to feed our family nutritious homemade meals from whole ingredients without breaking the bank. That makes this recipe my go-to, Monday night, need-something-on-the-table-quick-that-everyone-will-love recipe. I use only a pound of grass-fed ground beef but pack it with nearly 6 cups (800 g) of 5 different vegetables! This recipe sure isn't fancy, though I'll bet it's the one that gets made regularly.

Serves 2 to 4

2 to 3 tbsp (30 to 45 mL) bacon grease, lard or coconut oil

1 cup (150 g) diced onion

1 cup (175 g) diced zucchini

1 cup (175 g) chopped bell pepper

½ cup (100 g) diced carrots

2 cups (200 g) chopped kale

1 tsp (5 g) kosher salt

1 lb (454 g) grass-fed ground beef

3 cloves garlic, minced

1 batch Taco Seasoning Blend (here)

Preheat a large skillet or heavy-bottomed pan to medium and melt your desired fat. I prefer lard and bacon grease to coconut oil in this dish flavor-wise, but coconut is so good for you, it would still be fine to use if you are accustomed to the flavor.

Add the onion, zucchini, bell pepper, carrots and kale to the hot pan along with the kosher salt. Cook and stir until the vegetables are almost tender, about 7 to 9 minutes.

Dump the par-cooked vegetables in a large bowl and set aside. Return the pan to the heat and add a tablespoon (15 mL) of additional fat if the pan has dried out at all. When the pan is back up to temp at medium heat, cook the ground beef, garlic and Taco Seasoning Blend until the beef is browned, 10 to 12 minutes. This may look like a lot of seasoning, but it is meant to also flavor the vegetables. It's going to be the right amount for the overall dish.

When the ground beef is nearly done, return the par-cooked vegetables to the pan and continue cooking together for another 5 minutes, or until the vegetables are fully cooked. (Hint: Judge this by the doneness of the carrots. They're the veggie that will take the longest.) Serve right away or divide into storage containers for premade protein to be used within the next 5 days.

TIP: Ultimate Taco Meat can be used in so many ways and is an excellent recipe to include in your weekly food prep. I love to reheat some to put over leafy greens with fresh guacamole for an easy weekday lunch. You'll love this recipe!

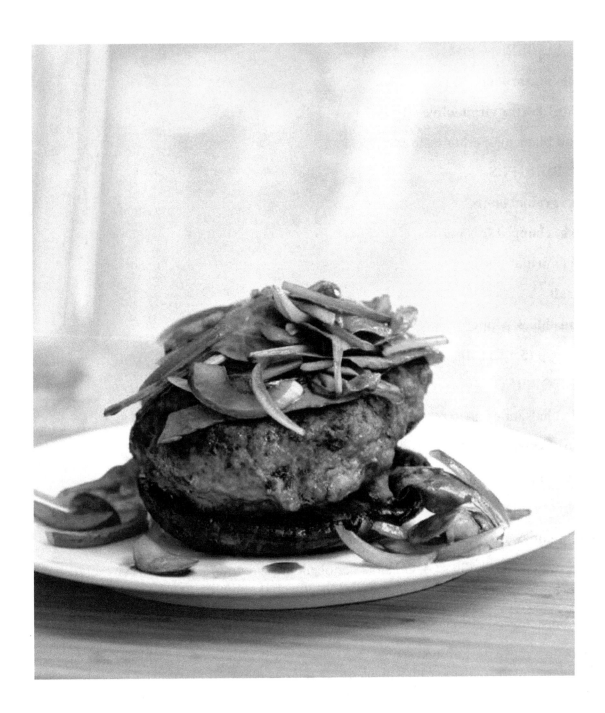

OPEN-FACED GREEK SLIDERS

From the roasted portobello "bun" to the crown jewel of fresh and tangy salad, there is no question that you are in for triple layers of flavor! This is how you make fancy food like lamb taste fantastic for a fraction of what you'd spend on the premium cuts. Pair this bold dish with Mushroom Diavolo (here) and Zoodles with Chilies and Vinegar (here) for a first-round TKO against bland meals.

Serves 4

FOR THE SLIDERS

4 portobello mushrooms

1 tbsp (15 mL) extra virgin olive oil

Sea salt and black pepper, to taste

FOR THE BURGERS

1 lb (454 g) ground lamb

¼ cup (10 g) chopped fresh mint

1 tsp (5 g) paprika

½ tsp sea salt

6 to 7 grinds black pepper

Optional: 1 tsp (5 mL) extra virgin olive oil, if cooking burgers on the stovetop

FOR THE TOPPING

1 tsp (5 mL) balsamic vinegar

2 tsp (10 mL) extra virgin olive oil

Pinch of sea salt

1 cup (38 g) organic baby spinach

4 (¼ inch [6 mm]) slices red onion (cut in half to make strips, not rings)

Preheat the oven to 400°F (204°C). Grab the portobello mushrooms and clean off any dirt using a dry kitchen towel. Resist the temptation to wet the towel. If you were to use a wet towel, the mushroom would absorb the moisture like a sponge; resist. Start from the top center of the cap and gently brush toward the outer edge. That's it.

Use a spoon to remove the gills and stems, then lightly brush both sides of each cap with the olive oil and season the gill side with a pinch of sea salt and a few grinds of black pepper. Lay the portobellos gill side up on a baking sheet lined with foil, parchment or a silicone mat. Roast for 20 minutes, turning them over once at the 10-minute mark.

When the portobellos are finished roasting, take them off the baking sheet and place them on a serving dish to await their burger counterparts.

While the mushrooms are roasting, combine all of the ingredients for the burgers thoroughly by hand and divide into 4 equal sections. Shape into patties and set aside.

The burgers can be grilled or cooked on the stovetop in a skillet. For the grill option, preheat the grill to at least 450°F (232°C) and place the lamb patties on the grate. Grill over direct heat for about 4 to 5 minutes per side for medium doneness. The same general rules apply for the stovetop, except add a teaspoon of extra virgin olive oil to the skillet so the burgers don't stick. Cook the burgers over medium-high heat for about 4 to 5 minutes per side.

Whether stovetop or grill, while the lamb burgers cook, dress the simple salad. Whisk the vinegar, olive oil and sea salt together in a small bowl. In another bowl, toss the baby spinach and red onion slices together. Drizzle with the vinegar mixture. Toss again to coat the salad with the dressing. Set aside.

Retrieve the burgers and place on the waiting roasted portobellos. Top each burger with a handful of fresh salad and serve fresh.

PÂTÉ FOR ROOKIES

Organ meats are little jewels in the Paleo world. Few items on your menu will contain as much nutrition per bite as kidney, heart and liver. Unfortunately, they are not always the most palatable options. Enter pâté. Pâté gives us the opportunity to season up liver and play with the texture a little bit. Since liver is on the bitter side, I've balanced that with the sweetness of nutrient-dense prunes. Trust me, it works. If you are new to pâté, or organ meats in general, give this one a try. This is the best pâté I've ever had!

Yields 1 cup (200 g)

½ cup (75 g) diced yellow onion

2 cloves garlic, minced

½ tsp dried thyme

6 prunes (about ⅓ cup [40 g])

1 tbsp (15 mL) apple cider vinegar

Pinch of red-pepper flakes

1 bay leaf

2 tbsp (30 g) ghee

8 oz (230 g) calf's liver, cubed

½ tsp coarse sea salt

6 grinds black pepper

In a large skillet over medium heat, cook the onion, garlic, thyme, prunes, vinegar, red-pepper flakes and bay leaf in the ghee, stirring often, until fragrant. Add the calf's liver along with the sea salt and pepper and cook for 4 to 5 minutes.

Remove and discard the bay leaf. Transfer the liver mixture to a food processor. Puree until completely smooth.

Transfer to an airtight container and chill in the refrigerator. Serve cold.

GROUND BEEF STIR-FRY WITH WILTED NAPA CABBAGE

There are times when I want the taste of stir-fry, but I don't want to mess with slicing and searing thin cuts of beef. Ground beef makes a great and affordable substitute! When it's piled on top of quickly prepared napa cabbage, a full meal hits my table in under a half hour.

Serves 4 to 6

---

2 to 3 tbsp (30 to 45 g) lard, bacon grease or coconut oil (see note)

2 lb (908 g) grass-fed ground beef

1 (8 oz [116 g]) can sliced water chestnuts

½ cup (75 g) sliced bamboo shoots, cut into matchsticks

1 inch (2.5 cm) fresh gingerroot, peeled and cut into matchsticks

4 cloves garlic, minced

¾ cup (177 mL) coconut aminos

Pinch of black pepper

2 tbsp (20 g) sesame seeds, plus

1 tsp (4 g) for garnish

1 head napa cabbage, sliced across the grain

½ cup (25 g) thinly sliced green onions

This stir-fry comes together quickly since both components of the meal—the ground beef and the napa cabbage—cook simultaneously. For some of you, that's good news. For others, it might come across as confusing. I'll break the directions down into separate pans and you decide if you want to wing them at the same time or prep the ground beef first, then move on to the cabbage.

Ground beef pan: Heat a skillet over medium-high heat and melt 2 tablespoons (30 g) of your preferred fat from above. Add the ground beef and begin to cook. After about 5 to 6 minutes, when the beef is halfway done, add the water chestnuts, bamboo shoots, ginger and 3 cloves of the minced garlic. Cook until the meat has completely browned, another 5 minutes or so. Add ½ cup (118 mL) of the coconut aminos, a pinch of black pepper and 2 tablespoons (20 g) of the sesame seeds. Simmer for 7 minutes, or until most of the coconut aminos have reduced.

Napa cabbage pan: Heat a skillet over medium heat and add 1 tablespoon (15 g) of your preferred fat. Add the sliced cabbage, toss in the fat to coat and let wilt. When the volume is reduced by a third, add the remaining 1 clove of minced garlic and toss to evenly distribute. After about 10 minutes, or when the cabbage is nearly done, add the remaining ¼ cup (60 mL) of coconut aminos. Remove the pan from the heat as soon as the coconut aminos reduce slightly (another 5 to 6 minutes).

To serve, family style presents nicely. However, only about half of the ground beef "fits" over the napa. Layer the napa cabbage on a serving platter first, then spoon on the ground beef stir-fry. Top with the remaining 1 teaspoon sesame seeds and the green onions. As for the remaining beef, we just add extra onto our plates.

Note: If you choose not to use grass-fed beef, please scale back the amount of fat to only 1 tbsp (15 g). It will be very oily if you don't.

BALSAMIC ROSEMARY BEEF

Every now and again that glorious moment strikes when you see it: a sale on grass-fed steak. When, not if, opportunity strikes, pull this recipe out and enjoy a gourmet grilled steak; it's good for the soul. I like to keep a bottle of balsamic vinegar on hand for recipes like this where a little goes a long way. I don't mind spending a few extra bucks on a special ingredient so long as I'm able to get the most for my money.

Serves 3 or 4

---

3 cloves garlic

1 to 2 sprigs rosemary

1 tsp (5 g) coarse sea salt

¼ cup (60 mL) balsamic vinegar

¼ cup (60 mL) extra virgin olive oil

2 to 3 lb (908 g to 1.3 kg) beef steaks (whatever you can get a deal on)

For the marinade, mince the garlic cloves and chop the fresh rosemary first, adding them to a small mixing bowl in which the marinade will be combined. Fresh rosemary has an inedible stem, so the leaves will need to be removed prior to chopping. Hold the tip of the rosemary sprig in one hand and grip the stem with the other. Drag your fingers down the stem, removing all the rosemary leaves in the process. Discard the stems and chop the leaves. A tablespoon (about 5 g) is about right for this amount of beef.

Add the salt and vinegar to the mixing bowl. Then, while whisking, stream in the olive oil to create a well-incorporated emulsion of oil and vinegar.

Now onto the beef. From tri-tip to rib-eye, you never know what's going to go on sale. Thankfully, this marinade works great on anything. Put the steaks in a large resealable plastic bag and pour in the marinade. Seal securely with limited excess air in the bag and move the steak and marinade around until the steak is evenly and completely coated. Allow to rest for 20 minutes at room temperature. Room temperature steak is not only easier to impart flavor into, but it also cooks faster and more consistently than refrigerator-temp meat.

Preheat a seasoned grill to high or about 500°F (260°C). Lay the steaks down in a single, uncrowded layer and grill to desired doneness. Serve alongside Overnight Salad (here) and Hard Cider Sprouts (here)!

On Grilling Steaks …

Cook times will vary depending on the cut and desired doneness. However, there are a few cues to know if you are getting close. Generally, grilled meat is ready to turn when it easily lifts away from the grates. If the meat is clinging to the grill, it needs a little more time.

Thermometers obviously give an accurate read but piercing the steak to insert the thermometer will release the juices, draining the meat of moisture, which keeps it tender. There are infrared thermometers that can read temperature without disturbing the meat itself; however, they are costly, making them a less ideal choice.

Ultimately, the pressure test is the way to go. Pressing on the center of the steak to see how much resistance the meat gives can determine doneness—no purchase necessary! Hold your thumb to your pointer finger (making the "OK" symbol). Now touch the thick, fleshy portion of your thumb. As you hop from pointer to pinky, that muscle in your thumb will flex, giving you a scale on which to compare your steak. Each finger represents a point of doneness: medium-rare, medium, medium-well and well done—rare is when the thumb is held out (like you're giving a high five) and is not flexed or touching a finger. Ideally steaks are cooked at medium-rare to medium, so if your steak matches the feeling of the meaty part of your thumb when it presses your pointer or middle finger, you've arrived.

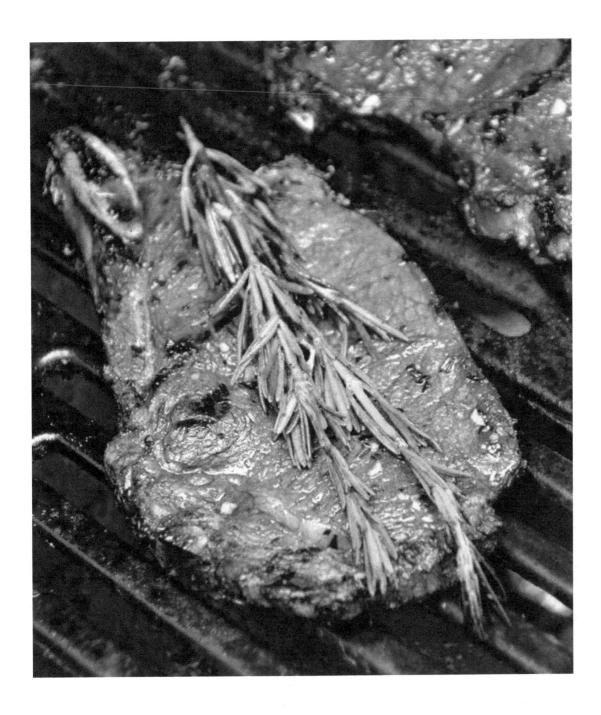

SLOW COOKER TACO SOUP

This is as minimal as taco soup gets—yet it is a favorite among my family and non-Paleo guests alike! These basic ingredients do a great job of creating a nutritious and easy taco soup, but feel free to jazz it up with your own ideas. Maybe toss in some sliced jalapeño or chipotle peppers for a spicy kick, or swap out the bell peppers for diced sweet potato for a stewlike version. The recipe is very flexible.

Serve with a dollop of Spinach Guacamole Salsa (here) or some diced avocado and fresh cilantro.

Serves 6 to 8

---

1 tbsp (15 g) Paleo-friendly fat, such as lard, bacon drippings, tallow or coconut oil

1 lb (454 g) grass-fed ground beef

2 to 3 cloves garlic, chopped

1 batch Taco Seasoning Blend (here)

1 tsp (5 g) kosher salt

3 organic carrots, chopped

2 bell peppers (red, yellow or orange), diced

1 small onion, diced

3 (14.5 oz [411 g]) cans fire-roasted diced tomatoes

In a large skillet over medium heat, melt your choice of fat. Add the ground beef, garlic, Taco Seasoning Blend and salt and par-cook for about 7 to 8 minutes. Par-cooking gives the ground beef a start but does not fully cook the meat.

Dump the seasoned ground beef mixture, including the residual fat and pan juices, into a slow cooker. Add the remaining ingredients, cover and cook on low for 4 to 5 hours.

LAMB MEATBALLS IN CREAMY CURRY SAUCE

While a rack of lamb can be intimidating, ground lamb is not. The price is just a touch more per pound than ground beef, and it's certainly a budget-friendly alternative to a pound of chops. These meatballs are blended with bold garlic and fresh parsley and gently simmered in a tomato-based curry sauce, finished with coconut milk. You'll hardly believe this entire meal runs less than $20 from start to finish.

Serves 3 to 4

FOR THE MEATBALLS

1 lb (454 g) ground lamb

2 cloves garlic, finely minced

1 tbsp (10 g) chopped fresh flat-leaf parsley

½ tsp kosher salt

6 to 7 grinds fresh black pepper

FOR THE SAUCE

2 tbsp (30 mL) extra virgin olive oil or coconut oil

½ medium white or yellow onion (about 3 inches [8 cm] wide), diced

3 cloves garlic, minced

1 tsp (5 g) kosher salt

1 (14.5 oz [411 g]) can crushed organic tomatoes

1 tbsp (15 g) curry powder (regular, not spicy)

½ cup (118 mL) full-fat, canned coconut milk

Chopped fresh mint, for garnish

Start by preparing the meatballs. In a large bowl, combine all of the ingredients listed for the meatballs by hand. Use a quarter-cup (60-mL) measuring cup (or anything comparable) to scoop out the mixture and shape into balls. This helps keep them uniform for even cooking time. There should be about 10 meatballs total.

Heat a Dutch oven or large heavy-bottomed pot with a secure lid over medium-high heat. Pour in the oil. When it comes to temp, arrange half of the meatballs in the pot without them touching each other. Leaving plenty of room in between the meatballs will allow the oil to stay hot, resulting in a quality sear on the meat. Sear the meatballs on at least 2 sides, then transfer to a bowl or plate (a paper towel to absorb fat is not necessary) and continue cooking until all of the meatballs are done.

In the same pot, add the onion, garlic and kosher salt and reduce the temperature to medium. Cook and stir until the onion becomes translucent, about 6 to 7 minutes.

Add the tomatoes and curry powder and allow to bubble. When the mixture just starts to bubble up a few times, reduce the temperature to low and return the meatballs to the pot. Mix the meatballs into the sauce, cover and simmer for 30 minutes.

At the 30-minute mark, remove the lid, turn off the heat and pour in the coconut milk. Stir until fully combined.

Transfer to a serving dish and top with chopped fresh mint or even some leftover fresh flat-leaf parsley, whatever is easiest and most accessible.

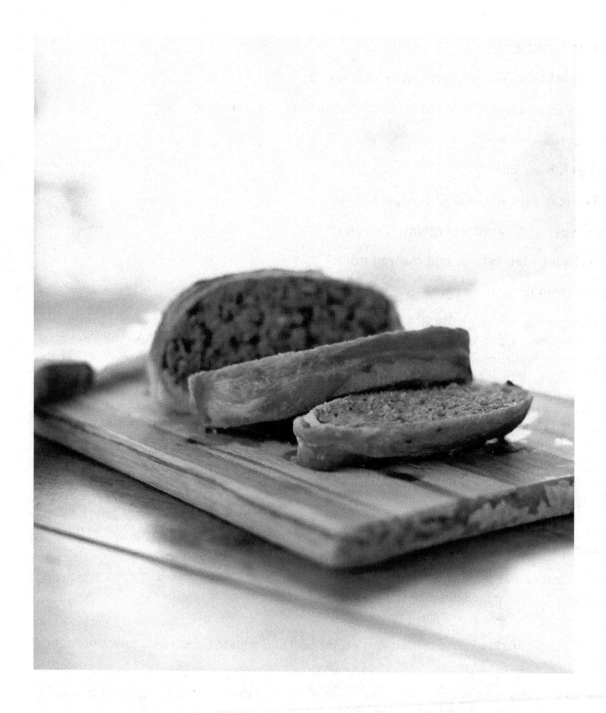

OFFAL BACON MEATLOAF

I should actually call it Offal GOOD Bacon Meatloaf! My favorite way for sneaking in food that isn't on the favorites list with my kids is to mix it in with ground meats such as meatballs and meatloaf. There is no way that I can get them to eat plain liver, but I can put a slice of this on their plates and get them to clean it. I suppose the bacon isn't hurting my cause either.

Serves 6 to 8

½ cup (120 g) Pâté for Rookies (here)

1 ½ lb (356 g) grass-fed ground beef

1 cup (100 g) finely chopped mushrooms

½ cup (75 g) finely diced onion

¼ cup (10 g) chopped fresh parsley

½ tsp dried thyme

½ tsp coarse sea salt

About 10 bacon slices (quality pastured bacon free of preservatives, sugar, gluten and nitrates)

Preheat the oven to 375°F (190°C). Grab the reserved batch of Pâté for Rookies (here) if you made it ahead of time. If not, prepare it now before moving to the next step.

In a large bowl, using your hands, combine the ground beef, pâté, mushrooms, onion, parsley, thyme and sea salt. Place on a baking sheet and form a loaf about 6 inches wide by 10 inches long (15 cm x 25 cm). Slice by slice, lay the bacon across the loaf, tucking the ends under each side to secure. Be sure the slices just barely overlap so there are no gaps in your wrapping. About 10 slices should cover the length of the meatloaf—just eyeball proportions as you work. If 10 slices aren't enough, grab a few more. If the meatloaf is covered in 7 or 8, reserve the other 2 or 3 slices for another recipe.

Bake for about an hour. You'll want to insert a meat thermometer into the center to be sure it has fully cooked. When the center of the meatloaf reaches 160°F (74°C), the beef is done. Remove the meatloaf from the oven and allow to rest for 5 to 10 minutes before slicing and serving.

If you have a good Paleo ketchup or BBQ sauce recipe, whip it up while the meatloaf cooks. It's a perfect sauce for dipping!

GREEN BEAN CASSEROLE WITH SWEET POTATO "ONIONS"

Casseroles are hard to come by in Paleo, so this recipe is a keeper. While it may not be a convenient mash-up of premade, processed foods like the category is known for, it does hit that perfect comfort food note using fresh, whole foods.

Serves 6 to 8

FOR THE "ONIONS"

1 (1.5 lb [681 g]) sweet potato (not yam)

2 tbsp (30 g) coconut oil, melted

1 tsp (5 g) onion powder

½ tsp garlic powder

½ tsp kosher salt

FOR THE CASSEROLE

1 batch Cashew Cream Sauce (here)

2 tbsp (30 g) coconut oil

½ lb (227 g) grass-fed ground beef

1 cup (75 g) white or cremini mushrooms, chopped

½ yellow or white onion, diced (about ¾ cup [100 g])

3 cloves garlic, minced

1 tsp (5 g) kosher salt

¼ tsp freshly ground black pepper

1 tsp (2 g) dried organic thyme

4 cups (600 g) fresh green beans, trimmed and cut into 1-inch (2.5-cm) pieces

If you'd like to top the casserole with the sweet potato "onions," make those first. Preheat the oven to 425°F (218°C). Meanwhile, peel the sweet potato and cut it into shoestrings either by using a spiral slicer or a julienne peeler. It's important the shoestrings not be too thick or they will not cook properly.

In a large bowl, toss the potatoes with the melted coconut oil. Then add the onion and garlic powders and toss again. Transfer to a baking sheet lined with either parchment or a silicone mat and bake for 20 minutes. Remove the baking sheet from the oven, mix up the potatoes and return to the oven to continue baking for another 5 to 7 minutes, or until the potatoes are fully cooked.

Sprinkle with the kosher salt and set the sweet potatoes aside for later.

Reduce the oven temperature to 350°F (177°C).

Be sure to have a full batch of Cashew Cream Sauce on hand first, then move forward preparing the casserole.

In a large, heavy-bottomed skillet, melt the coconut oil. Once the oil has melted, crumble the ground beef into the pan along with the mushrooms, onion, garlic and kosher salt, pepper and thyme. Cook for 9 to 11 minutes, or until the beef is nearly done, then add the trimmed green beans. Cook for another 7 to 8 minutes, or until the beef is fully cooked and the green beans have softened slightly.

Pour the prepared Cashew Cream Sauce into the ground beef mixture and simmer on low for about 5 minutes while you ready the casserole dish.

Select a large casserole dish, about 13 inches by 9 inches (33 cm by 23 cm) works for this amount of food. Pour the contents of the skillet into the casserole dish, cover with foil and bake for 20 minutes, or until the sauce is bubbling.

Remove from the oven, top with the reserved sweet potato "onions" if you made them, and serve warm.

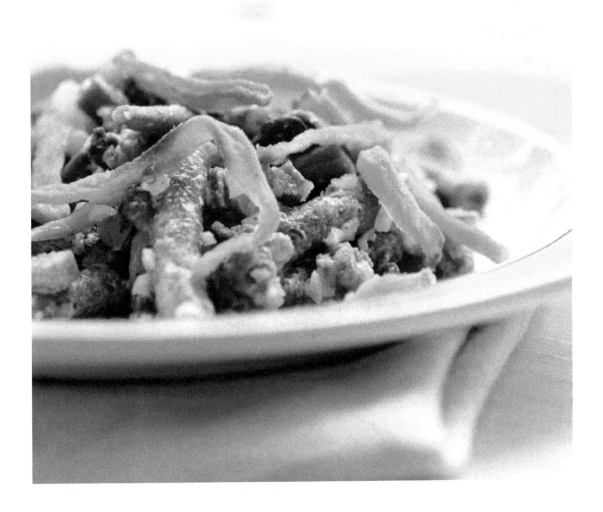

BRAISED SHORT RIB KEEMA

Keema is an Indian dish that is typically prepared with ground beef and peas. But I couldn't resist the opportunity to rub its bold seasonings on beef short ribs and give them a

slow braise. This dish goes great with some basic cauliflower rice and Kohlrabi "Papadum" Chips (here) on the side.

Serves 3 to 4

FOR THE SPICE BLEND

1 tsp (4 g) garam masala

1 tsp (5 g) kosher salt

½ tsp onion powder

½ tsp garlic powder

¼ tsp ground ginger

½ tsp ground coriander

½ tsp ground cumin

¼ tsp regular chili powder

FOR THE RIBS

2.5 to 3 lb (1.1 to 1.3 kg) beef chuck short ribs (about 5 or 6 pieces)

2 tbsp (30 g) ghee

1 cup (237 mL) beef stock

1 tbsp (15 mL) lemon juice

Chopped fresh cilantro, for garnish

Preheat a Dutch oven or large pot suitable for braising over medium-high heat. In a small bowl, blend together the dry spices to create a bold rub for the short ribs.

In a large bowl, toss the short ribs together with the spice rub, evenly coating all of the ribs.

Drop the ghee into the Dutch oven. When it melts, is glossy and slides easily over the bottom of the pan when tilted from side to side, add 2 or 3 spiced short ribs to the pan to sear. Sear each rib for about 4 minutes on each side, or until a nice golden crust forms. The meat does not need to be fully cooked-searing is the first step to braising the meat. Repeat until all of the ribs have been browned.

Return all of the ribs to the pan, pour in the beef stock and lemon juice and cover. Reduce the temperature to low and braise for 3 hours, or until the beef is fork-tender and falls away from the bone with little resistance.

Serve with freshly chopped cilantro sprinkled over the ribs and with that braising liquid nearby for dipping; it's delicious.

VEGETABLE BEEF CURRY

It doesn't always take a lot of ingredients to pull out some serious flavor. Just a few select spices paired with inexpensive stew meat (or cubed beef chuck) and a handful of veggies make this bold and easy one-pot dinner. And any dish that finishes on the stovetop or in the oven long enough for me to tidy up the kitchen afterward gets a bonus in my book.

Serves 2 to 4

---

1 tsp (5 g) ground turmeric

1 tsp (5 g) kosher salt

½ tsp curry powder

1 ¼ to 1 ¾ lb (567 to 794 g) cubed beef chuck (stew meat)

2 tbsp (30 g) ghee

1 cup (150 g) sliced carrots (½ inch [1 cm] slices)

1 cup (150 g) fresh green beans, trimmed

1 inch (2.5 cm) fresh gingerroot, peeled and julienned

2 cloves garlic, minced

1 cup (237 mL) beef stock

Fresh cilantro, for garnish

Start by preheating a Dutch oven or large heavy-bottomed pan suitable for braising to medium-high.

While the pan heats, create a quick spice rub with the turmeric, kosher salt and curry powder. Toss the cubed beef or stew meat in the rub, coating every little corner evenly.

Add the ghee to the pan and begin searing the cubed beef. Work in batches so the meat doesn't overcrowd the pan. Putting too many pieces of meat into the pan will drop the temperature to the point where it will no longer sear but steam the meat—not what we're going for right now. So divide up the meat based on the size of both the pan and the beef and sear away. Each piece of beef will need about 3 minutes per side to get a nice crust. The inside of the beef will remain undercooked at this point.

Once all of the beef has been seared, return it to the pot and also add the carrots, green beans, ginger and garlic. Mix together. Cook, stirring occasionally, for 3 to 4 minutes, or until the garlic and ginger are fragrant.

Pour in the beef stock and use it to scrape up the browned bits that have stuck to the bottom of the pan. This process is called deglazing.

Reduce the heat to low, cover and allow to braise for 30 minutes. At this point the beef will be just done and will have a steak-like texture. Garnish with cilantro. Whether served as a thick stew or alongside cauliflower rice, this exotic dish makes a great meal.

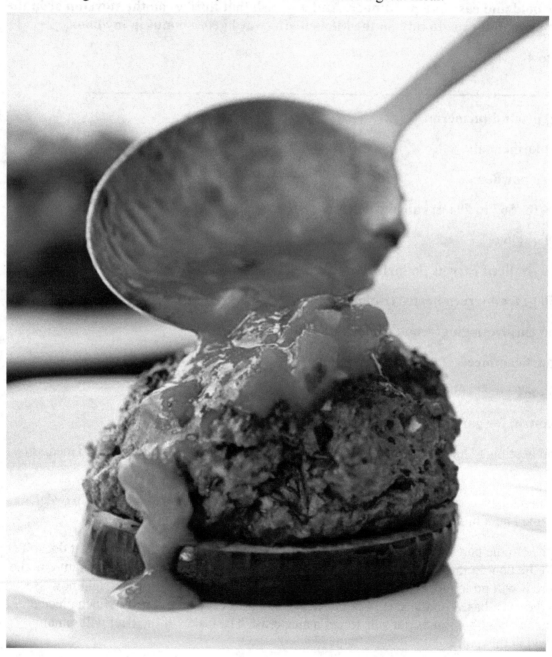

EGGPLANT SLIDERS

This dish was inspired purely out of a need to use up a leftover half eggplant and some ground beef that had been defrosted a few days prior. Dinner at my house can frequently

be compared to the Food Network's show *Chopped*. In this case, grass-fed ground beef patties seasoned with herbs and garlic lay atop thick eggplant steaks and are topped with a quick and zesty tomato sauce; it really works!

Serves 4

FOR THE SAUCE

¼ cup (60 mL) extra virgin olive oil

½ cup (75 g) diced yellow onion

2 to 3 cloves garlic, minced

½ tsp sea salt

½ tsp dried basil

Just barely ⅛ tsp cinnamon

Pinch of red-pepper flakes

1 ½ cups (356 mL) organic crushed tomatoes

1 cup (237 mL) organic chicken stock

FOR THE SLIDERS

1 lb (454 g) grass-fed ground beef

¼ cup (10 g) chopped fresh flat-leaf parsley

1 clove garlic, minced

1 tsp (3 g) dried basil

½ tsp kosher salt

1 tbsp (15 g) coconut oil, lard, bacon drippings or another Paleo-friendly fat

FOR THE EGGPLANT

4 (½ inch [1 cm]) slices eggplant

A drizzle of extra virgin olive oil

A dusting of House Seasoning Blend (here)

Pinch of kosher salt

Chopped fresh flat-leaf parsley or basil, for garnish

While the ingredients list may appear extensive, it's really just the same items used in the three different elements that make up the full recipe. The base is a seasoned thick eggplant steak, which is topped by an herb and garlic grass-fed burger and then finished with a quick marinara.

Start by getting the marinara on to simmer. Classic, dare I say **correct**, tomato sauce has a touch of cinnamon in it. This may be new to some of you, but trust me, you will appreciate the depth it provides. Heat a saucepan over medium heat with the olive oil. When the oil comes to temp, add the onion and garlic and cook and stir until they have softened a bit, about 5 to 7 minutes. Then add the sea salt, basil, cinnamon and red-pepper flakes. Mix and simmer for only a minute or less, then add the crushed tomatoes and chicken stock. Stir it up, cover and reduce the heat to low. Simmer away while the other components are prepared.

Next, preheat the oven to 400°F (204°F); this is for the eggplant later. Also, preheat a large skillet to medium-high on the stovetop (this is for the burgers).

With your hands, thoroughly combine the ground beef with the parsley, garlic, basil and kosher salt. Divide into 4 equal portions and shape into patties.

Melt the coconut oil (or your choice of fat) in the preheated skillet and sear the seasoned beef patties. The burgers do not need to be fully cooked, just crusted on each side. Sear for about 4 minutes, or until the burgers are browned.

While the beef sears, lay the eggplant slices in an ungreased baking dish, drizzle with olive oil and dust with House Seasoning Blend and a pinch of kosher salt. Only do this for 1 side.

To bring the Eggplant Sliders together, lay a burger patty on each eggplant slice and top each with a heaping quarter cup (60 mL) of cooked tomato sauce. Loosely cover the dish with foil and bake for 15 to 20 minutes.

After removing the sliders from the oven, garnish with a little chopped fresh flat-leaf parsley or basil and eat with a knife and fork.

CREOLE-STYLE MARROW

In Paleo, we prize gelatin and fats sourced from grass-fed animals, making beef marrow an absolute treasure. This recipe takes advantage of marrow's richness by adding savory Creole seasonings and finishing with bright lemon and parsley. Who needs bread? Grab a spoon and enjoy!

Serves 2 to 4

---

1 batch Creole Seasoning Blend (here)

1 pound (450 g) small or medium grass-fed beef marrow bones

1 tsp (5 g) coarse sea salt

1 lemon, quartered

¼ cup (10 g) chopped fresh flat-leaf parsley

Preheat the oven to 450°F (230°C).

Combine the ingredients for the Creole Seasoning Blend from here.

Place the marrow bones in a large bowl and sprinkle the seasoning blend and sea salt over the bones, tossing to evenly coat.

Arrange the bones standing up on their ends in a roasting pan large enough to allow a couple of inches/several centimeters between their neighbors. The bone is essentially the serving vessel when it comes to marrow, so we want to do our best to keep it contained. Laying them on their sides will let all of that marrowy goodness melt out of the bone and onto your roasting pan. That's not what we want. Keep them standing upright. Roast for 20 to 25 minutes.

The marrow is done when it has melted and started pulling away from the bone. It may even bubble up a little bit. Remove from the oven and transfer the bones to a serving dish.

To finish, squeeze fresh lemon juice over the tops and sprinkle with the parsley. Allow the bones to cool slightly before handling. Then, using a small spoon or even a butter knife, reach down into the bone and lift out the marrow, bite by decadent bite. Reserve some fresh lemon for additional squeezing as you work your way into the bone, if you prefer.

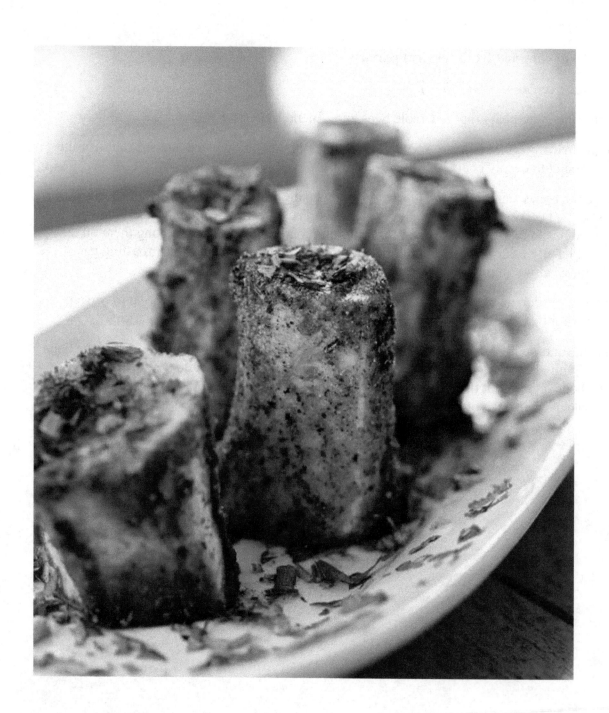

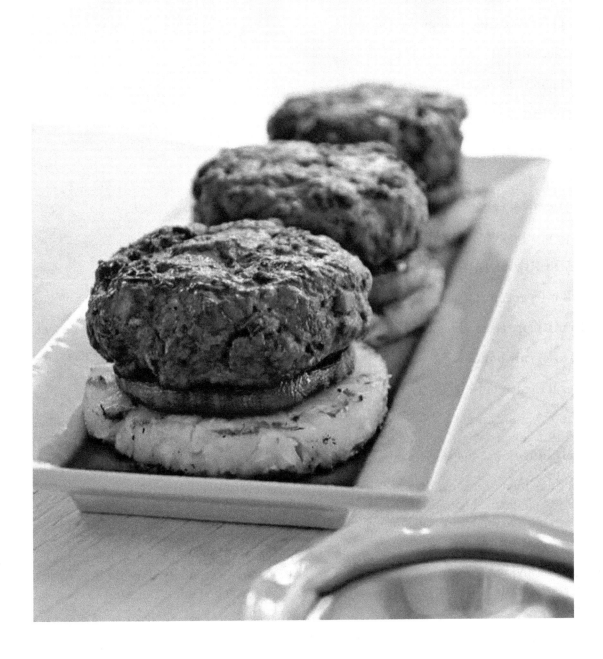

TERIYAKI STACKERS

Our family loves burgers! But just a single patty on a plate is boring. Let's stack on the flavor—literally. Lightly grilled red onion and thick pineapple slices under a grass-fed burger packed with classic Asian ingredients—plus a quick and easy 3-ingredient teriyaki sauce on the side for dipping—make each bite a mouthful of anything but boring.

Serves 4

1 lb (454 g) grass-fed ground beef

1 tbsp (15 g) finely diced jalapeño

1 clove garlic, minced

2 tbsp (5 g) chopped cilantro

½ tsp kosher salt

1 tsp (4 g) sesame seeds

½ tsp onion powder

4 (½ inch [1 cm]) slices fresh pineapple

4 (¼ inch [6 mm]) slices red onion

FOR THE TERIYAKI DIPPING SAUCE

½ cup (118 mL) coconut aminos

1 tbsp (15 mL) rice wine vinegar or coconut vinegar

¼ cup (60 mL) raw honey

Preheat a grill to medium-high heat.

First, mix together the burger patties and get them on the grill. In a large bowl, by hand, combine the ground beef, jalapeño, garlic, cilantro, kosher salt, sesame seeds and onion powder. Divide into 4 equal portions and shape into patties.

Grill the burgers to your desired doneness alongside the fresh pineapple and red onion slices. I like to grill the pineapple and onion for just 2 to 3 minutes per side, just to get the char marks but not enough to change them much, texturally speaking.

While the grill is going, mix up the quick teriyaki dipping sauce. In a small bowl, combine the coconut aminos and vinegar, then stream in and whisk the honey to emulsify. Portion the dipping sauce into equal amounts for the number of people you'll be serving and hold at room temperature.

Grab the burgers, pineapple and onion off the grill. Stack the pineapple slices, then the onion slices and then the burgers on your plates or serving tray and serve alongside the teriyaki dipping sauce. Eat these with a knife and fork, making sure to get each layer in every bite!

POOR MAN'S BRACIOLE

Traditional braciole rolls a filling of bread crumbs, Parmesan and often Italian sausage into a large flank steak, which is then oven-roasted or braised to finish. It's delicious but not Paleo-friendly. It can also be a bit of an investment, both financially and time-wise, to prepare. Here's an alternative to costly flank steak using grass-fed ground beef! It is filled

with nutrient-dense, Paleo-friendly ingredients and cooks easily in the oven for a budget-friendly, gourmet Italian main course.

Serves 6 to 8

FOR THE BEEF

2 lb (908 g) grass-fed ground beef

¼ cup (28 g) coconut flour

1 batch Italian Seasoning Blend (here)

1 tsp (5 g) kosher salt

1 egg

FOR THE FILLING

Extra virgin olive oil

4 cups (152 g) sliced organic baby spinach

½ cup (75 g) diced yellow onion

2 cups (138 g) chopped white mushrooms

3 cloves garlic, minced

Pinch of kosher salt and black pepper

Preheat the oven to 375°F (190°C) and prepare the beef.

In a large bowl, combine the beef, coconut flour, Italian Seasoning Blend, salt and the egg by hand until thoroughly mixed together. Let this rest while the filling is prepared.

Heat a sauté pan or skillet to medium-high and drizzle in a few tablespoons (about 30 to 45 mL) of extra virgin olive oil—enough to lightly coat the bottom of the pan. When the oil is hot (is glossy and slides easily across the pan when tilted from side to side), drop in the spinach, onion, mushrooms, garlic and kosher salt and pepper. Cook until the spinach has wilted, the mushrooms have softened and the onion is translucent, about 7 minutes. Remove the pan from the heat and allow the filling to cool slightly during the next step.

Turn the seasoned ground beef out onto a clean work surface lined with either parchment paper or a silicone mat. Use a rolling pin to roll the ground beef into a quarter-inch (1-cm)-thick rectangle—about 14 inches by 9 inches (36 cm by 23 cm). This "sheet" replaces the flank steak.

Spoon the slightly cooled vegetable filling onto the flattened ground beef, leaving a 2-inch (5-cm) edge at one narrow end of the beef (the short 9-inch [23-cm] side). Leaving a section of beef without filling will help to secure the beef to itself once it is rolled up.

Use the parchment paper or silicone mat to help "jelly roll" the beef, starting from the end with the filling and working toward the end without. I recommend rolling the beef a half to full turn, then giving the log a small squeeze to secure, much like how sushi is rolled. Continue with this process until the end of the beef is reached. Press the section of "unfilled" beef into the roll to secure the log, then use the parchment paper or silicone mat to carefully transfer the braciole to a baking sheet or large roasting pan. If your pan isn't nonstick, you may want to cook the braciole on top of the parchment or silicone sheet to avoid sticking. If your pan is nonstick, the paper or silicone sheet is not necessary. In any event, be sure the braciole is placed seal side down.

Bake for 45 minutes, or until the internal temperature of the braciole reaches 160°F (71°C). Allow the beef to rest for 10 minutes or so before slicing, so the juices have a chance to redistribute back into the meat, ensuring juicy meat instead of a "juicy" cutting board.

This is great served with your favorite marinara sauce alongside roasted spaghetti squash or even just some simple green beans, sautéed kale or chard, or Pan-Roasted Cauliflower and Zucchini (here).

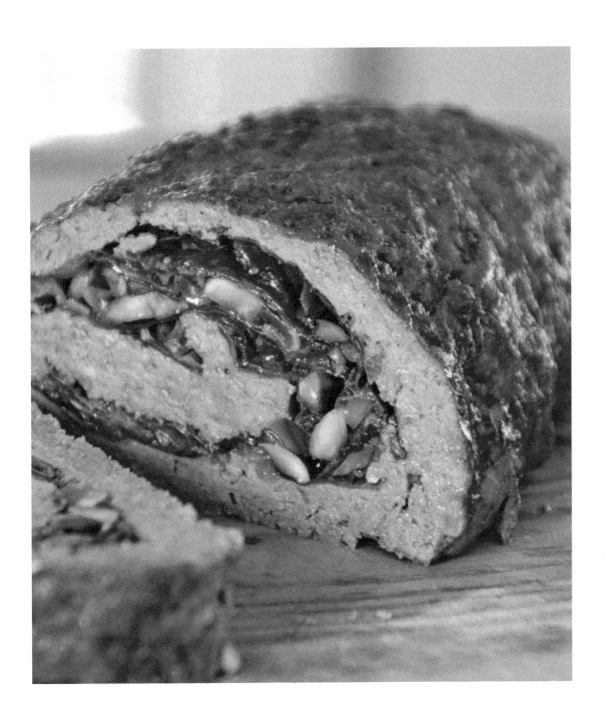

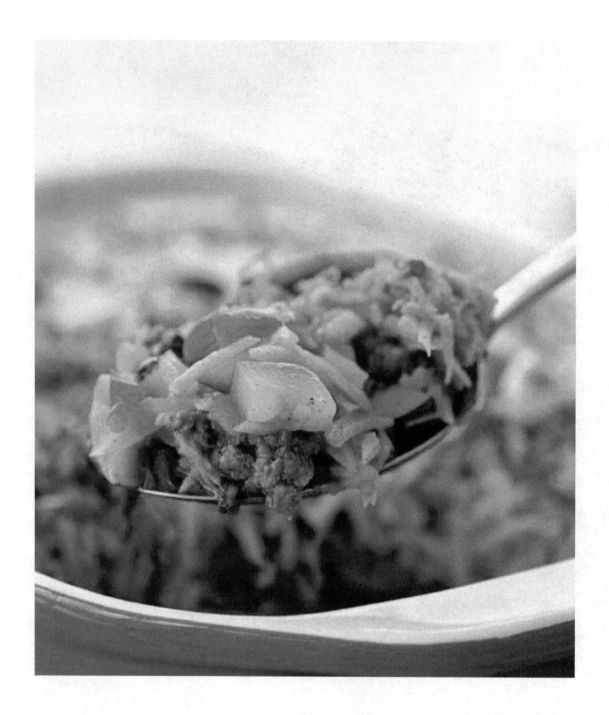

TEX-MEX CASSEROLE

This is a favorite on my blog, Popular Paleo. I think it's so well liked not just because casseroles are hard to come by in Paleo, but because it's loaded with affordable vegetables that stretch the pound or so of grass-fed ground beef. You can feed a table full of hungry guests for just a few bucks a head. And by the way, these leftovers make an awesome breakfast when reheated and topped with a runny fried egg. Grab your favorite hot sauce and enjoy this delicious meal that pulls double duty.

Serves 6 to 8

3 tbsp (45 g) preferred Paleo-friendly fat (bacon drippings or lard, preferred)

2 cups (76 g) organic baby spinach

2 to 3 organic carrots, diced

1 medium yellow onion, diced

1 (6 inch [15 cm]) zucchini, diced

2 cups (350 g) diced bell peppers

3 to 4 cloves garlic, minced

½ tsp sea salt

1 to 1 ½ lb (454 to 683 g) grass-fed ground beef

1 batch Taco Seasoning Blend (here)

1 (14.5 oz [411 g]) can organic diced tomatoes

FOR THE SWEET POTATO TOPPING

3 large sweet potatoes or yams

½ cup (115 g) coconut oil

½ tsp onion powder

½ tsp chili powder

½ tsp ground coriander

Fresh cilantro, sliced green onions, avocado and hot sauce, for garnish (optional)

Preheat the oven to 375°F (190°C).

In a very large skillet or heavy-bottomed pan over medium heat, melt 1 tablespoon (15 g) of your chosen fat and add in the spinach, carrots, onion, zucchini, bell peppers and garlic. Season with the sea salt, stir and cook until the vegetables are just about fork-tender, about 10 minutes. Remove from the pan and set aside for later.

In the same pan, add the remaining 2 tablespoons (30 g) of fat and get it up to temp. Crumble in the ground beef, top with the Taco Seasoning Blend and stir to combine. Cook until the beef browns, about 10 to 12 minutes.

While the ground beef browns, grate enough sweet potatoes or yams to yield 5 cups (750 g). Dump them in a large mixing bowl.

Melt the coconut oil and pour over the shredded sweet potatoes while it's warm. Toss immediately. The coconut oil will start to solidify again as it cools, so work efficiently. Once the sweet potatoes and coconut oil are mixed well, sprinkle them with the onion powder, chili powder and coriander. Mix together.

Add the cooked vegetables plus the diced tomatoes back into the pan with the beef. Mix carefully to bring everything together and cook for about 3 minutes—just to let all of the ingredients get to know each other for a second. Transfer all of this veggie-meaty goodness to a 13 inch by 9 inch pan (33 cm by 23 cm) or other large casserole dish. Top with the seasoned, shredded sweet potatoes, cover with foil and pop in the oven.

Bake for 20 to 30 minutes, then remove the foil and broil on low for about 5 minutes, or until the sweet potatoes have browned and crisped up a bit; eyeball it.

To serve, top with fresh cilantro and sliced green onions with some avocado and hot sauce on the side.

PALEO HOTDISH (A.K.A. TATER TOT CASSEROLE)

Traditional Hotdish, or Tater Tot Casserole, this is not. Leave your expectation for a pool of processed foods at the door and instead prepare yourself for a whole lot of fresh vegetables and budget-friendly grass-fed ground beef—the heart of the Paleo plate.

Serves 6 to 8

---

2 tbsp (30 mL) extra virgin olive oil

1 cup (150 g) diced carrots

½ cup (50 g) diced celery

1 cup (100 g) diced parsnips

Pinch plus 1 tsp (5 g) kosher salt

1 medium (3 inch [8 cm]) white or yellow onion, diced

3 cloves garlic, chopped

1 cup (100 g) chopped mushrooms

2 lb (908 g) grass-fed ground beef

2 recipes Classic Ranch Seasoning (here)

1 (14.5 oz [411 g]) can organic cut green beans, drained

One recipe Sweet Potato Tater Tots (here)

1 tsp (5 g) nutritional yeast (optional)

Preheat the oven to 375°F (190°C).

Start preparing the casserole by heating a large, high-sided skillet to medium-high and adding the olive oil. When the olive oil has come to temp (is glossy and slides easily across the pan when tilted from side to side), add the carrots, celery, parsnips and a pinch of kosher salt (no more than a quarter teaspoon). These denser veggies need a head start on the other ones. Cook and stir for about 10 minutes, or until they soften. (Note that the temperature is kept so high because the pan will be quite crowded, constantly challenging the pan to maintain a heat that can efficiently cook this volume of food.)

Add the onion, garlic, mushrooms, ground beef, all of the Classic Ranch Seasoning and the remaining 1 teaspoon (5 g) kosher salt. Take time to break down the ground beef into crumbles and mix all of the ingredients together until evenly combined. Cook and stir for another 13 to 15 minutes, then add the drained green beans and stir into the mixture. Finish cooking for another 3 to 4 minutes, then transfer to a deep baking or casserole dish, about 11 inches by 8 inches (28 cm by 20 cm).

Top the meat and veggies with a single layer of prepared Sweet Potato Tater Tots and bake for 20 minutes, uncovered. If you like to use nutritional yeast, sprinkle about a teaspoon (5 g) of it over the beef and vegetables prior to adding the tater tot layer.

Allow to cool for 5 minutes before serving.

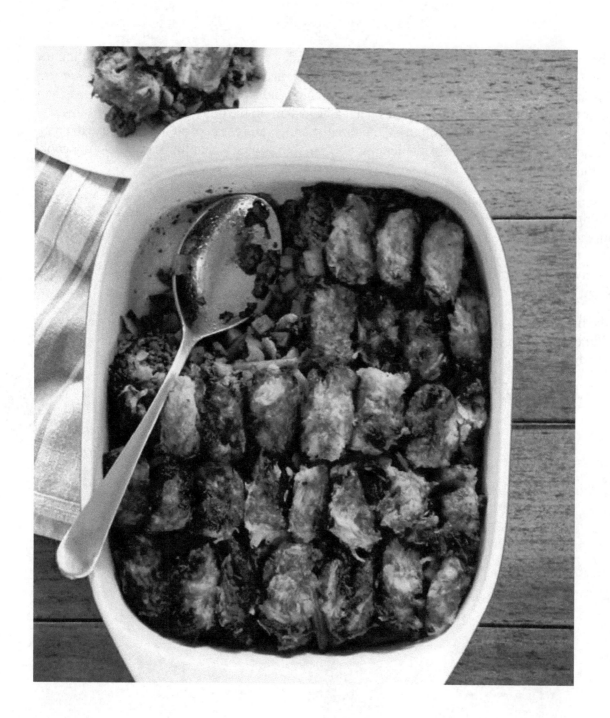

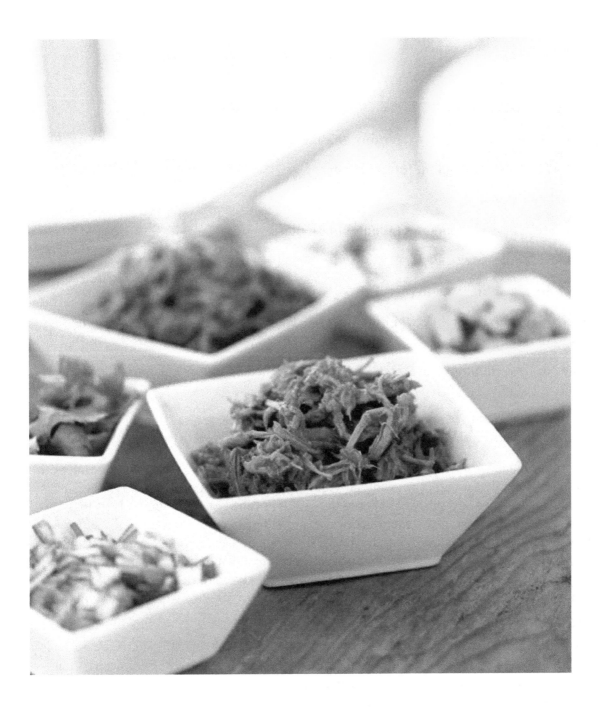

BARBACOA

Traditional barbacoa looks little like what you're likely to come across in eateries nowadays since most of us are not partial to the cuts that compose the authentic dish. And while authenticity has its place, practically speaking many of us are looking for creative yet approachable dishes we can incorporate into our regular meal rotations. Barbacoa sounds fancy, but really it is just an inexpensive cut of beef with some spices and a few vegetables.

Serves 6 to 8

2 lb (908 g) grass-fed beef chuck

1 batch Fajita Seasoning Blend (here)

1 tsp (5 g) kosher salt

2 tbsp (30 g) Paleo-friendly fat, preferably animal-based

1 medium white or yellow onion, thinly sliced

3 cloves garlic, crushed

1 lb (454 g) fresh organic tomatoes (about 5 to 6), diced

2 tbsp (30 mL) apple cider vinegar

2 cups (514 mL) beef bone broth (here)

Chopped fresh cilantro, a squeeze of lime juice, diced avocado, sliced radishes and/or finely diced red onion, for garnish

Prepare the beef by trimming away excess fat and gristle, then cutting into 3- to 4-inch (8- to 10-cm) cubes.

In a large bowl, combine the spices to make one batch of Fajita Seasoning Blend plus the kosher salt. Add the cubed chuck to the bowl and toss with the spices until evenly coated.

Break out your Dutch oven or favorite pot for braising and preheat it to medium high. Melt your choice of Paleo-friendly fat in the pan and grab your favorite pair of tongs. When the fat is hot, use the tongs to arrange a few pieces of beef in the bottom of the pot, being careful not to overcrowd. Attempting to sear too many pieces at once will drop the temperature of the pan, resulting in steaming rather than searing the meat. Not what we want here. So work in batches, allowing for about an inch (2.5 cm) of space between each piece in order to get that crispy, golden sear. Sear all sides of the meat, then transfer to a clean bowl to rest. If the pan looks a bit dry after browning the beef, add another tablespoon or so (15 to 30 g) of whatever fat you used before. Reduce the temperature to medium.

For the braising liquid, add the onion and garlic to the hot pan; cook and stir. When the garlic is fragrant and the onion is translucent, add the diced fresh tomatoes and the apple cider vinegar. When the juices begin to bubble, return the beef cubes to the pot and nestle them into the tomato sauce. Cover with the broth, gently move the meat around to mix the ingredients slightly, and wait for the braising liquid that you've just made to bubble up once more.

When the braising liquid begins to boil, reduce the temperature to low to keep it from boiling during the braising time and cover the pot with a secure lid. Braise the beef for 2 hours, or until the meat is tender and gives little resistance when pressed on with the back of a spoon or fork. If additional time is necessary, check every 15 minutes until the right texture is achieved.

To finish the beef, remove it from the liquid and shred by hand. Discard any large pieces of fat and gristle.

To finish the sauce, bring the braising liquid to a boil (uncovered) and reduce the liquid by half, which should take about 7 to 10 minutes. When the liquid becomes a thickened sauce, reserve 1 cup (237 mL) of concentrated tomato and onion first, then puree the remaining sauce using an immersion blender, high speed blender or food processor. Return the puree, the reserved cup of thickened braising liquid and the shredded beef to the pot and combine.

Serve on top of roasted portobello mushrooms, in large lettuce leaves or spooned over cauliflower rice for a Mexican-style burrito "bowl." I like to top this with chopped fresh cilantro, lime juice, diced avocado, sliced radishes and finely diced red onion.

STUPID EASY ASIAN BEEF

This recipe is an ode to one of my favorite people and bloggers, Stephanie of Stupid Easy Paleo. Since her favorite meat and veggie combo is beef and asparagus, this recipe is for her. Make it in the summer when asparagus is in season and reap the savings on a tasty Asian-inspired one-dish dinner.

Serves 4 to 6

---

2 lb (908 g) top sirloin (or another inexpensive cut of steak)

1 tbsp plus ¼ cup (15 mL plus 60 mL) coconut aminos

1 lb (454 g) fresh asparagus

1 to 2 green onions

3 cloves garlic

½ cup (65 g) raw cashews

Lard, coconut oil or avocado oil (the fat for this recipe must be able to tolerate high cooking temperatures)

¼ tsp kosher salt

½ cup (118 mL) beef bone broth (here)

Toasted sesame seeds and/or chia seeds (optional)

Start by preparing the beef. It needs to be sliced fairly thin, which can be done easily with partially frozen meat. Either work with steak that is partially defrosted or place your steak in the freezer for about an hour to firm up.

Identify which direction the grain of the steak is going and situate the meat so that when sliced, it is across the grain and not alongside it. Taking the time to slice the steak across the grain will yield a more tender piece when cooked, which is particularly important since the beef is flash fried. If you stretch the steak back and forth like an accordion and see lines rather than circles, you're cutting in the wrong direction. Rotate the steak a quarter turn and try again.

Slice all of the steak and place in a medium mixing bowl. Mix 1 tablespoon (15 mL) of the coconut aminos into the beef to subtly season. Set aside to rest at room temperature while the other ingredients are prepared.

While the beef rests, trim the dried ends of the asparagus first and discard them. Slice the stalks into 1-inch (2.5-cm) segments on the bias (cut diagonally). Cut the green onions in the same fashion, thinly sliced on the bias. You should get about 2 to 3 tablespoons (15 to 23 g). Discard the white ends of the green onions. Mince the cloves of garlic and roughly chop the raw cashews.

Now that all of the ingredients are chopped, sliced and minced, it's time to quickly bring the dish together. The hardest part is behind you.

Heat a large skillet or wok to medium-high and add 1 tablespoon (15 g) of selected fat to the pan. Be sure to choose a pan with a broad base as opposed to a narrower bottom, since narrower pans will force all the meat into a pile, making it difficult to sear.

When the fat is glossy and moves easily across the pan, arrange a few of the steak slices in a single layer. (Do not crowd). Sear 1 side, then transfer to a separate bowl for temporary holding. Searing takes less than 3 minutes, so this step will move quickly. Repeat the searing process until all of the steak is cooked. Should the pan dry out and need additional fat between batches, by all means add it. Work 1 teaspoon (5 g) at a time, a batch at a time until all of the steak has been seared.

In the same pan, add another teaspoon (5 g) or so of fat and allow it to come to temp. When it is glossy and moves easily across the pan, quickly add the asparagus, garlic and kosher salt. Stir-fry for 2 to 3 minutes, then deglaze with the beef bone broth and the remaining ¼ cup (60 mL) coconut aminos. Deglazing is a process that lifts all of the browned bits from the bottom of a hot pan by the addition of liquid. The liquid and heat work together to dissolve those browned bits and turn them into flavor gems, adding richness and depth to any pan sauce.

When the pan has fully deglazed, which usually takes just 2 to 3 minutes, return the reserved beef to the pan with the vegetable mixture and combine. Reduce the temperature to medium and continue to cook and stir for 5 to 7 minutes. When the broth reduces by half, add the green onions and cashews and combine.

Transfer to a serving dish. If desired, top with either toasted sesame seeds, chia seeds or both.

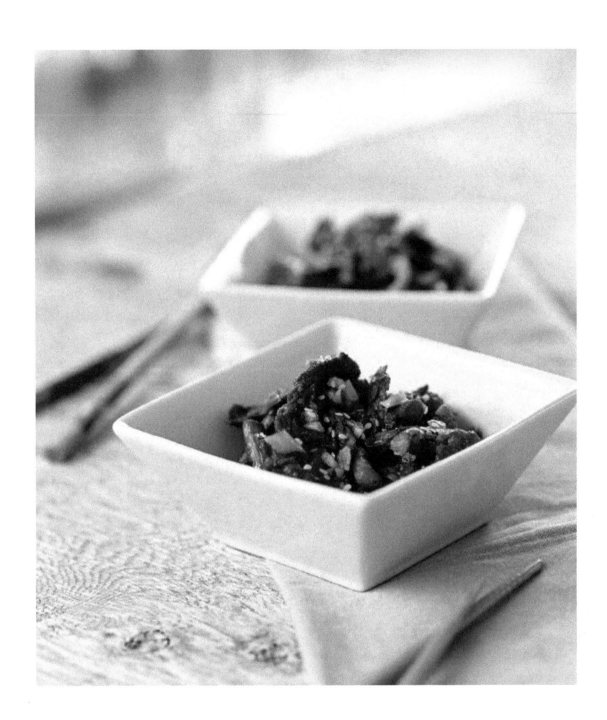

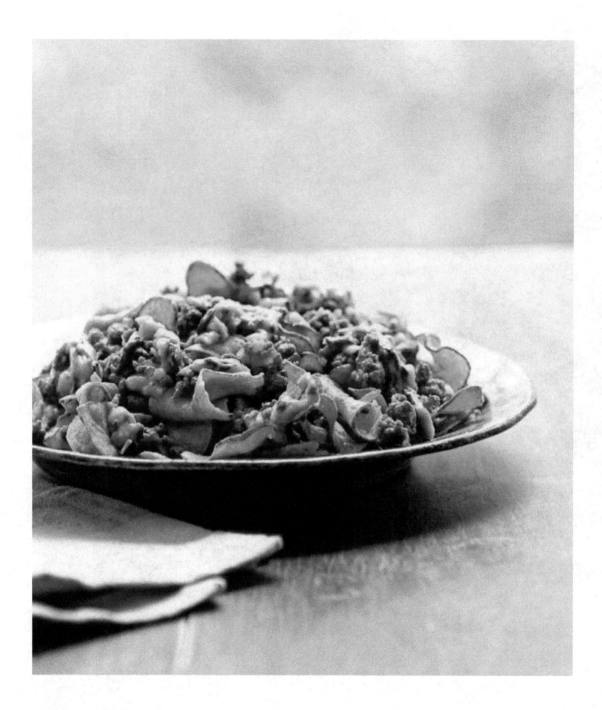

IRISH NACHOS

Irish Nachos use fries or homemade thick-cut potato chips in place of tortilla chips and are usually loaded with melted cheese and spicy taco meat. For the Paleo version I like to pack this recipe with nutrient-dense fixings like Spinach Guacamole Salsa and Ultimate Taco Meat. It's a crafty way to turn junk food into health food. *You're welcome.*

The trick to quality Paleo Irish Nachos is in the chips. Now, frying thin-cut sweet potatoes in a cup or so of your choice of fat isn't exactly the most cost-effective way to prepare homemade chips, though they certainly are quite reliable and tasty that way. The most cost-effective method to get this job done is with the oven. Unfortunately, the trick for getting oven-baked sweet potato chips crispy is a multistep process. If you are able to find suitable premade sweet potato chips, then by all means, please do so. But if you've ever wanted to knock those chips out from scratch, this is how to do it.

Serves 2 to 4

---

2 lb (454 g) yellow sweet potatoes (not orange yams)

1 batch Ultimate Taco Meat (here)

1 batch Spinach Guacamole Salsa (here)

Pinch of sea salt

It's common to think that the secret to getting the chips crisp is hot and fast cooking, but that's actually not ideal. Baking at a lower temperature for a slightly longer time frame draws out the moisture in the sweet potatoes without bothering the natural sugars, so we end up with a golden brown, dry and crispy chip as opposed to a partially burnt, yet still mysteriously soggy slice of sweet potato.

The first step is to bake the sweet potatoes in a preheated 400°F (204°C) oven for only 30 minutes. This will be long enough to soften the potatoes, but not get them to the texture of baked potatoes that you'd have as a side dish with some coconut oil and sea salt. Bake the potatoes for 30 minutes and allow to cool completely before moving to the next step. The potatoes can be held overnight in the refrigerator if you'd like to make this process more convenient by dividing it into stages.

Preheat the oven to 300°F (149°C) and peel the cooled sweet potatoes. Use a mandoline slicer or a steady hand and sharp knife to thinly slice the potatoes.

Lay the slices in a single layer on a parchment-lined baking sheet. Bake for 30 minutes, then turn the slices over and continue baking for an additional 30 to 35 minutes. The chips should be a light golden color at this point.

Remove the chips from the oven, sprinkle with a pinch of sea salt and allow to cool completely before moving to the next step. Cooling the chips is a critical step—this is where the crispness sets in. Don't skip it.

To assemble the Irish Nachos, prepare a batch of Ultimate Taco Meat and a batch of Spinach Guacamole Salsa. Of course, it's best to have prepared these items in advance. However, they can also be prepared alongside the crispy sweet potato chip process if you are comfortable multitasking in the kitchen. Reheat the Ultimate Taco Meat if it is not already warm.

On a large serving tray, lay out the fresh sweet potato chips and top with Ultimate Taco Meat. Spoon the Spinach Guacamole Salsa into a large resealable plastic bag, seal and snip off a corner to create about a ¼-inch (6-mm) opening. Pipe the salsa onto the meat to finish off the nachos. Serve immediately.

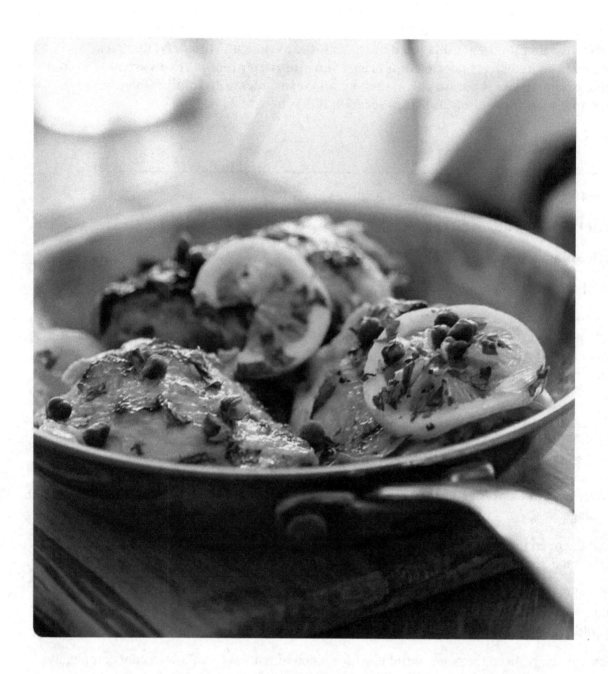

Chicken seems to be the protein folks love to hate. It's been called boring, bland, overpriced (for the boneless, skinless varieties) and "gross" when you have to break down the whole bird yourself. Ouch. Can't a bird catch a break?

I mean, think of a protein that is as depended upon as chicken….

Having guests to dinner? Chicken.

Exhausted after a long day? Chicken.

On a budget? Chicken.

Let's face it, chicken is the vanilla ice cream of the protein world. It's the blank slate we can't seem to get away from. So embrace it by making the most out of every bird.

As a mom of two making this Paleo thing work on a single income in a semi-Paleo family, I rely on chicken to make Paleo-friendly meals that fool my biggest critics (you know, the hungry little ones sitting at my dining room table) as well as to stretch a dollar. After all, chicken rolls from meal to meal better than any other protein. Being "vanilla" has its advantages.

We can bounce from Asian-inspired dishes like Easy Thai Coconut Chicken (here) and Orange Cashew Chicken (here) to Mexican themes with Spatchcock Cilantro Lime Chicken (here) and Chicken and Chorizo Meatballs (here) before coming back around to homestyle favorites like Bacon Ranch Chicken (here) and Triple-Pepper Lemon Chicken (here). That's a good start to your meal planning right there!

But beyond tasty and diverse dinners, the real winner for me is what I can do with a roasted bird, such as with Roasted French Countryside Chicken (here). A typical life cycle of whole organic, free-range chickens looks like this in our home:

STEP 1: Roast two whole chickens.

STEP 2: Serve one as a meal; remove the meat from the bones on the other. Save the carcasses from both birds.

STEP 3: Use the reserved meat from the second chicken to premake chicken salads and breakfast skillets and to set aside for post-workout recovery protein or midafternoon munchies.

STEP 4: Make chicken stock from scratch using the saved bones.

All of this food will have the utmost nutritional benefits and is free of harmful chemicals that come from industrialized, non-organic chickens. When you consider how much was provided from two little birds, suddenly that price tag for organic free-range versus the commercial discount option doesn't seem so outrageous.

TRIPLE-PEPPER LEMON CHICKEN

This ain't your mama's lemon chicken! Blackening Seasoning Blend (here) combines black, white and cayenne peppers for a kick that will wake up anyone who rolls their eyes at yet another grilled chicken dish. This is unmistakably spicy, perfectly crisp and impeccably finished with a squeeze of fresh lemon while hot off the grill. This may sound gourmet, but it's as simple as grilling a few pieces of chicken. And speaking of chicken pieces, many grocery stores sell precut whole chickens for about the same cost as whole ones, so look around. You'll save yourself some time, too, buying chicken this way.

Serves 4

_____

1 whole organic, free-range chicken (about 4 pounds [1.8 kg]), cut into sections

1 batch Blackening Seasoning Blend (here)

½ tsp kosher salt

1 lemon, halved

Get the grill going so the temperature hits high heat, around 500°F (260°C).

Butcher your chicken into sections, or purchase one already cut up (which is how I like to do it). Toss the pieces into a large resealable plastic bag and sprinkle in the Blackening Seasoning Blend and kosher salt. Seal the bag tightly and toss to completely coat the chicken in the seasonings.

Place the chicken on the hot grill, reduce the heat to medium and close the lid. Let the magic of the grill do its work. Leaving the chicken as undisturbed as possible equals a quality cooking experience, which results in crispy, blackened chicken that is still juicy and moist.

After about 8 to 10 minutes, open the lid and turn the chicken. Close the lid again and cook for another 10 to 12 minutes.

At this point, check the internal temperature of the breast. The breast is the thickest section of meat on the grill, so if it is fully cooked, then the other pieces will be, too. Insert a meat thermometer from the side of the meat (not the top) and slide it into as close to the center of the breast as possible. The chicken is done when it reaches 165°F (74°C).

If the chicken requires more time on the grill, turn the pieces so the least-done side is down regardless of which side was cooked first. Always grill with the cover closed. Check the same piece of chicken in the same spot (so the chicken isn't overly punctured with thermometer holes, which lets critical juices escape from the meat) until the temperature reaches 165°F (74°C).

Remove from the grill, squeeze the juice from the lemon all over the chicken pieces and let rest for 5 minutes before serving.

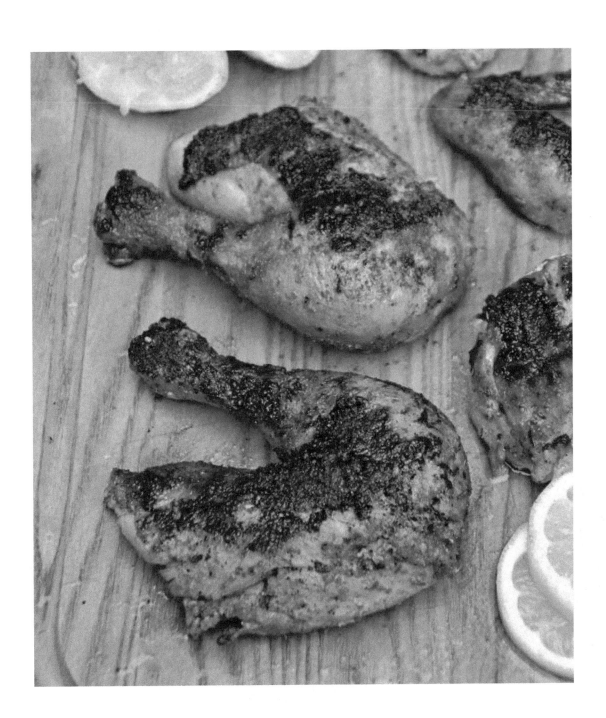

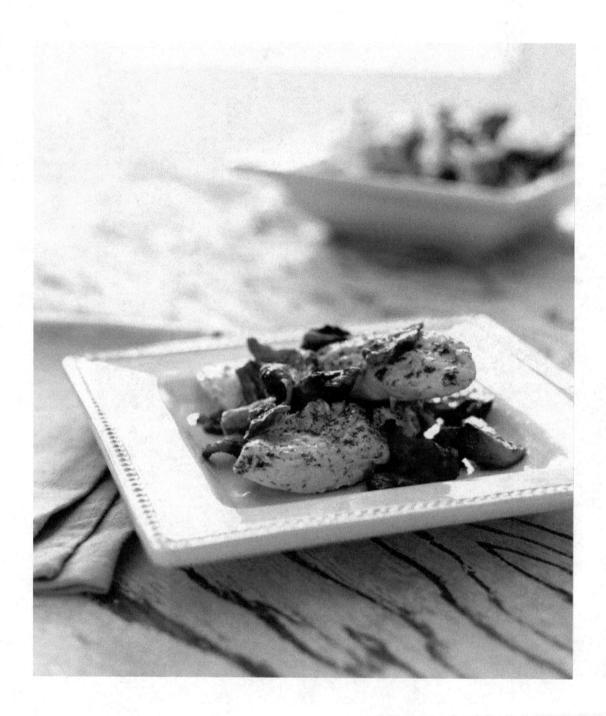

BACON RANCH CHICKEN

I made this dish with the intention of using up leftover bacon and mushrooms that I had in the fridge along with some chicken breasts (from a bulk purchase) I had taken out of the freezer a couple days prior. It turned out great! You'll love this recipe because it is cheap to make, finishes in the oven (which gives us a chance to clean up the kitchen before we sit down to dinner) and can be made start to finish in just about 30 minutes, depending on the cut of chicken used.

Serves 4

2 pounds boneless, skinless chicken breasts or thighs

2 tbsp (30 mL) extra virgin olive oil

1 tsp (5 g) kosher salt

1 tbsp (15 g) Classic Ranch Seasoning (here)

3 to 4 thick slices bacon, chopped (about 1 cup [225 g])

6 large white mushrooms

Chopped fresh flat-leaf parsley, for garnish (optional)

Preheat the oven to 375°F (190°C).

Trim the chicken of excess bits of fat and place them in a resealable large plastic bag. If you are using chicken breasts that exceed 3 inches by 6 inches (7.5 cm by 15 cm), cut them in half lengthwise so they will cook faster. If you are using thighs, just toss them in as is.

Add the olive oil, kosher salt and the Classic Ranch Seasoning to the bag. Seal and smoosh everything around so the chicken is evenly coated.

Place the seasoned chicken in a nonstick baking dish and bake, uncovered, for 30 minutes (for thighs) to 45 minutes (for breasts), or until the internal temperature reaches 165°F (74°C).

Next move on to the bacon and mushrooms. We're going to caramelize the mushrooms in the fat rendered from the bacon.

Toss the chopped bacon in a skillet or thick-bottomed sauté pan. Heat the skillet to medium and allow it to come to temp with the bacon.

While that's heating up, use a dry towel to clean the mushrooms. Start from the top of the cap and wipe toward the stem (going with the grain) to clean off any dirt left on the mushroom. Don't run them under water or they will soak it right up like a sponge. A dry towel does the trick!

Remove the stems and chop the mushrooms into bite-size pieces. We're not mincing here, just getting our 'shrooms into manageable bites.

When the bacon is about half done—meaning some fat has been rendered and the meat has firmed up a bit, but it's still considered undercooked—add the chopped mushrooms to the pan and mix together. Cook, stirring occasionally, for about 15 minutes, or until the bacon begins to crisp and the mushrooms caramelize.

When the chicken reaches 165°F (74°C), remove it from the oven and transfer the pieces to a serving dish. Top with the bacon and mushrooms and garnish with a little chopped fresh parsley, if desired.

TIP: Make it a complete meal by steaming some broccoli while the bacon and mushrooms are cooking!

CHICKEN AND CHORIZO MEATBALLS

Meatballs are one of those items that become a go-to protein in Paleo. They are incredibly adaptable and fast cooking. They are also super affordable. A triple threat! What's the catch? Unless you're a creative cook, they can get a little boring. Next time you find yourself in a meatball rut, break out this bold, spicy and unforgettable combination of ground chicken and quality pork chorizo. I like to have these with some sliced bell peppers and Easy Avocado Lime Salad (here) on the side for lunch.

Serves 3 to 4

---

12 to 16 oz (340 to 454 g) ground chicken

12 to 16 oz (340 to 454 g) quality pork chorizo

½ cup (75 g) finely diced red onion

1 large jalapeño, seeded and finely diced

1 clove garlic, minced

¼ cup (7 g) chopped cilantro

½ tsp kosher salt

1 egg

Preheat the oven to 400°F (204°C).

In a large bowl, combine all of the ingredients thoroughly by hand. It may take a few minutes to work everything together, but be sure that you do.

Use a quarter-cup measuring cup or something comparable to ensure equal scoops of the meatball mixture. Working one meatball at a time, scoop out some of the mixture, shape into a ball and then arrange on a baking sheet lined with parchment or a silicone mat. Be sure that there's at least an inch or so (2.5 cm) in between each meatball so all sides cook evenly.

Bake for 25 to 30 minutes, or until the internal temperature reaches 170°F (77°C). Serve hot.

OVEN-ROASTED JERK CHICKEN

It's been said that you cannot have enough roasted chicken recipes, and I have to say that I fully agree. I found that once I got the hang of roasting a whole chicken, it became a go-to meal for my family. Now I have fun mixing up flavors, like this recipe using spicy jerk seasoning. Classic jerk seasoning contains Jamaican allspice—a native berry that's dried and ground, much like peppercorns. If you've purchased this spice in the past, then you're likely looking for ways to use it again. This roasted chicken is just the thing!

Serves 4

---

1 whole organic, free-range chicken (about 4 pounds [1.8 kg])

1 small (2 to 3 inches [5 to 8 cm]) white or yellow onion

1 tbsp (15 g) Jerk Seasoning Blend (here)

1 tsp (5 g) kosher salt

1 tbsp (15 mL) coconut oil (grass-fed butter or ghee may also be used)

Preheat the oven to 400°F (204°C).

In general, a few things need to be taken care of before seasoning and roasting the bird. First, be sure to remove the gizzards from inside the cavity. Usually they are packed in a small bag, but that's not always the case—and it's not a guarantee all the little bits were caught. You'll want to remove the bag, plus any leftover bits still stuck to the walls of the cavity, and then give the chicken a rinse with cool water—inside and out.

Next, be sure to pat the outside of the chicken dry after the rinse and remove any quills or feathers what were missed during processing.

Now you have a few choices to make in terms of the wing tips and any excess skin around the base of the chicken located between the drumsticks. Personally I prefer to leave the wing tips in place and tuck them behind the back of the bird, though some do remove them with a knife. When it comes to the excess skin, I choose to remove it by trimming with a paring knife close to the cavity opening. Discard these items if removed or reserve and use later when preparing homemade chicken stock.

Most chickens have the necks removed, but in the event that yours does not, it should be trimmed prior to roasting. To do this, use a large knife to cut along both sides of the spine until you reach what is essentially the shoulders of the chicken. Grab the neck bone with one hand to secure it and, with the other hand, cut across the bone to sever the neck from the spine. The bird is now ready for seasoning.

Grab a small white or yellow onion, which will serve as our aromatic. When it comes to roasting poultry, an aromatic flavors the bird during the roasting process from the inside. Slice the onion in half from root to tip. Trim both ends and peel. Slice in half once more to quarter the onion into wedges and stuff inside the chicken cavity.

For the seasoning blend, mix together the dry spices, plus the kosher salt, and set aside.

Melt the coconut oil (or grass-fed butter or ghee) and coat the skin of the chicken, prioritizing the breasts, thighs and drumsticks. Set the chicken on a roasting rack or inside a roasting pan breast side up and pinch by pinch sprinkle the jerk seasoning evenly over the skin. Be sure to get into all the nooks and crannies. It's fine if seasoning falls into the pan as you work. It will mix with the juices as the chicken roasts and act as an aromatic.

After washing your hands, grab some butcher's twine and tie up the drumsticks, or "truss," to seal off the onion inside the chicken. This will ensure that all of the flavor from the onion steams directly into the meat, infusing it with even more flavor.

Bake the seasoned chicken uncovered for 1 ½ hours. Remove from the oven and let it rest at room temperature for 10 minutes prior to carving so the internal juices have enough time to redistribute back into the meat instead of running out all over your chopping block.

After 10 minutes have passed, transfer the chicken to a cutting surface and carve as desired.

BRAISED CHICKEN FAJITAS

Bell peppers are a key ingredient for fajitas, though they can be pricey if not on sale. Save some money by using a package of organic mini sweet peppers instead. They are often much more affordable for the same volume. Braised Chicken Fajitas is a near hands-free recipe that feeds my hungry family a filling dinner and still leaves enough for lunch leftovers the following day.

Serves 6 to 8

Paleo-friendly fat such as lard, tallow, duck fat, avocado oil or coconut oil

4 cups (700 g) red bell or mini sweet pepper slices, ½ inch (1 cm) thick

1 large onion, cut into ¼-inch (6-mm) slices

4 cloves garlic, crushed

1 batch Fajita Seasoning Blend (here)

1 tsp (5 g) kosher salt

1 whole bay leaf

1 cup (237 mL) organic, gluten-free chicken stock

1 pound (454 g) boneless, skinless chicken thighs and/or breasts

Heat a Dutch oven or large pot suitable for braising over medium-high heat and melt the selected Paleo-friendly fat. Be sure to choose a fat that can handle high temperatures. Lard from pastured pigs, duck fat, avocado oil or coconut oil are my preferences for this recipe.

Add the peppers, onion and garlic and cook, stirring frequently, until the onion becomes translucent and the garlic is fragrant, about 5 to 7 minutes.

Add the Fajita Seasoning Blend, kosher salt and bay leaf to the vegetables. Continue to cook and stir for another 2 minutes—enough time to draw out moisture from the vegetables that the pan deglazes (all the brown bits are lifted from the bottom of the pan and it appears "clean"), but not so long that the pan begins to get "dirty" again.

Pour in the chicken stock and bring to a boil. No need to adjust the temperature; the stock will boil at medium-high.

Tuck the chicken pieces into the stock and veggies so they are mostly submerged, then cover the pan with a secure lid. Reduce the temperature to low or to a temperature that will allow the stock to bubble without becoming a rolling boil. Braise for about an hour, or until the chicken shreds easily, but the peppers have not overcooked and become mushy. Remove and discard the bay leaf.

Remove the chicken from the braising liquid, shred and return it to the pot. Bring the liquid to a boil once again and cook, uncovered, until the liquid reduces to your preferred amount. For example, if you would like to eat this as a soup, topped with fresh avocado, cilantro and sliced radishes, then you may not want to reduce the liquid at all. However, if you would like to make a "burrito bowl" by serving the chicken fajitas over cauliflower rice (see here), topped with diced tomatoes and guacamole, then you may want to reduce the liquid quite a bit.

Here's an idea! To really stretch this meal, do a combination of the two. Spoon out your desired amount of shredded chicken, peppers and onion and serve over cauliflower rice, wrapped in lettuce leaves or folded up in your favorite Paleo tortilla for the first meal. Then for a second meal, serve the remaining chicken and vegetables as a fajita soup with the topping ideas listed above.

CHUNKY GARDEN CHICKEN CACCIATORE

By now you're likely aware that *cacciatore* means hunter in Italian, indicating that Chicken Cacciatore is prepared "hunter style," or rustic. But what kind of Paleo practitioner would I be if I didn't represent the gatherers among us? Fresh vegetables cut into hearty chunks balance this dish to create likely the most definitive hunter-gatherer meal one can serve.

Serves 4 to 6

---

1 organic, free-range chicken (about 4 pounds [1.8 kg]), cut into 6 sections

Kosher salt and black pepper, to taste

2 to 3 tbsp (30-45 mL) extra virgin olive oil

8 oz (200 g) mini sweet peppers, quartered into chunks

½ medium (3 inch [7.5 cm]) white or yellow onion, diced

4 oz (125 g) mushrooms, quartered

3 cloves garlic, chopped

1 batch Italian Seasoning Blend (here)

1 tsp (5 g) kosher salt

2 ½ pounds (1.2 kg) fresh organic tomatoes, diced

Chopped fresh parsley or basil, for garnish (optional)

Heat a Dutch oven or large heavy-bottomed pot with a lid suitable for braising over medium-high heat.

Season the chicken pieces liberally with kosher salt and black pepper. Add the olive oil to the preheated Dutch oven. When the oil is hot (is glossy and moves easily in the pan when tilted from side to side), drop in the chicken, seasoned side down, to sear. Allow an inch or so (a few centimeters) in between each piece for even cooking. Cook until the skin is a crispy golden brown, then remove from the pan and set aside. Note that depending on the size of your pan and chicken, it may be necessary to work in batches to avoid overcrowding. Adding too many pieces of chicken to the Dutch oven will drop the overall temperature, resulting in steaming the chicken as opposed to searing.

In the same pan, drop the peppers, onion, mushrooms and garlic along with the Italian Seasoning Blend and salt. Cook until the vegetables are seared, about 2 to 3 minutes. Once vegetables are charred slightly, add the diced tomatoes, which will effectively deglaze the pan and create the braising liquid at the same time. Simmer for about 5 minutes.

Return the seared chicken to the Dutch oven and nestle in between the vegetables. Reduce the temperature to low, cover the pot and let braise for 30 minutes, or until the internal temperature of the breast meat is 165°F (74°C).

Turn off the burner and let the cacciatore rest for 15 minutes. (This is a great opportunity to prepare a light vegetable side dish). Serve family style, garnished with chopped parsley or basil, if desired.

ORANGE CASHEW CHICKEN

This takeout favorite is quite simple to make at home. Defrost some boneless, skinless chicken breasts or thighs (or a combination of the two) from your freezer, and in less than half an hour, dinner will be on the table. Serve this chicken with a batch of basic cauliflower rice or a Paleo-friendly pasta alternative such as shirataki, kelp or sweet potato noodles to round out that Asian takeout meal taste—minus the "junk food hangover" the next day.

Serves 4 to 6

FOR THE SAUCE

½ cup (118 mL) water

Zest from 1 orange

1 cup (237 mL) fresh squeezed orange juice

¼ cup (60 mL) coconut aminos

½ tsp ground ginger

⅛ to ¼ tsp crushed red-pepper flakes

2 tbsp (15 g) arrowroot powder

FOR THE CHICKEN

1 tbsp (15 g) Paleo-friendly fat; coconut oil, lard, duck fat or avocado oil preferred

2 pounds (908 g) boneless, skinless chicken breasts, thighs or a combination

Kosher salt, to taste

½ cup (60 g) whole raw cashews

¼ cup (15 g) thinly sliced green onions

1 tsp (3 g) toasted sesame seeds (optional)

It's best to start by preparing the sauce first, so the chicken can be quickly dressed once it has fully cooked. In a saucepan, combine all of the sauce ingredients except for the arrowroot powder and bring to a gentle boil over medium-high heat. Whisk well to fully incorporate the ground ginger and ensure there are no clumps. Once the sauce bubbles, turn off the heat and whisk in the arrowroot powder to thicken. Cover the pan and leave it on the warm burner while the chicken is prepared. (Remember to keep the burner off while it rests.) Be sure to give it a quick stir a few times while it waits to help maintain the right texture.

For the chicken, heat a large skillet to medium-high heat and add your selected Paleo-friendly fat. Allow it to melt as the pan comes to temp.

In the meantime, cut the chicken into bite-size pieces. Season with a heavy pinch of kosher salt. When the skillet reaches medium-high, place the chicken pieces in the pan in a single layer to sear. Leave the chicken undisturbed for 3 to 5 minutes, or until it lifts easily off the bottom. Turn the pieces and continue to cook, stirring occasionally, until the chicken is no longer pink and the juices run clear. This should take approximately 5 to 7 minutes.

When the chicken is done, drain any excess juices from the pan first, then pour in the orange sauce and add the cashews. Toss the chicken and cashews in the sauce until evenly combined and simmer over medium heat to thicken the sauce again—this should take only 3 minutes. Finally, transfer everything from the pan to a serving platter and top with the sliced green onions and toasted sesame seeds, if you'd like.

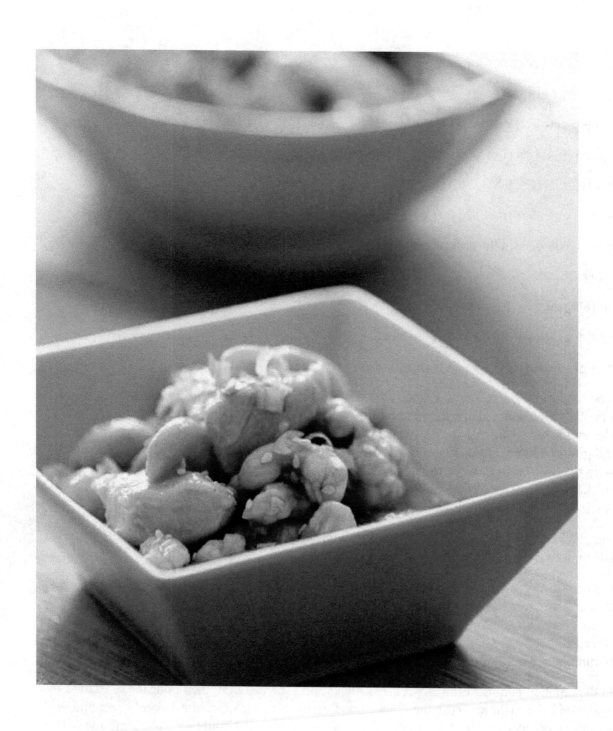

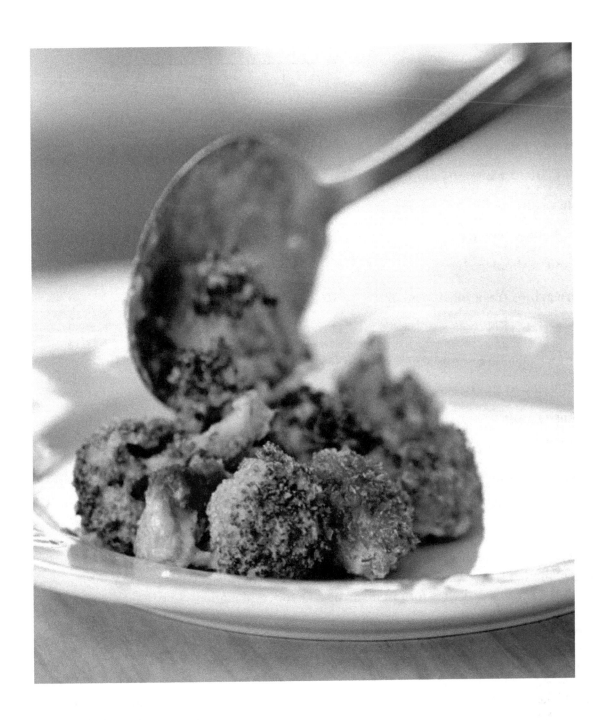

SKILLET CHICKEN DIVAN

There's something about a creamy chicken recipe that everyone loves. Chicken Divan is one of those classic casseroles with a canned cream-of-something soup base, chicken, ham and broccoli, smothered in cheese and uniquely seasoned with curry powder. However, it doesn't have to be that way! This Paleo version hits all the right notes thanks to a batch of Cashew Cream Sauce; it's no wonder it has been one of my top blog recipes for more than a year now.

Serves 4

FOR THE SAUCE

1 batch Cashew Cream Sauce (here)

2 cloves garlic, minced

1 cup (150 g) diced white or yellow onion

½ tsp kosher salt

1 ½ tsp (8 g) curry powder

½ tsp ground coriander

A few more grinds fresh black pepper

FOR THE CHICKEN

1 pound (454 g) boneless, skinless chicken breasts or thighs

1 tbsp (15 g) lard or your preferred Paleo-approved fat

Pinch of kosher salt

Fresh black pepper, to taste

2 cups (460 g) broccoli florets

¼ cup (25 g) flaxseed meal (optional)

Start by preparing the sauce. Follow the directions for a batch of Cashew Cream Sauce from here and incorporate the additional ingredients listed above required for this recipe. Essentially, you are taking a "mother sauce" and modifying it specifically for this dish. Once you get comfortable with this method, you can do this for just about any flavor combination! So while preparing the sauce, before the cup (237 mL) of chicken stock is streamed in, pulse the garlic and onion with the cashews to break them up, too. Then add the spices from the list above (kosher salt, curry, coriander and black pepper) and puree as the stock is added. The curry sauce for the Chicken Divan is now ready! Set it aside and move to cooking the chicken.

Chop the chicken into large, bite-size pieces. If using thighs, you can just leave them whole. I make this with both thighs and breasts and definitely prefer the whole pieces of thigh meat.

Heat a large skillet over medium-high heat and add your chosen fat.

Once it is hot (is glossy and slides easily across the pan when tilted from side to side), add the raw chicken and season with a pinch of kosher salt and a couple grinds of pepper. Stir occasionally and cook until the meat takes on a golden color, then dump the fresh broccoli florets onto the chicken—don't mix. Cover the pan and reduce the temperature to medium low. The broccoli should steam like this for 3 to 4 minutes, or until lightly steamed but still crunchy.

Grab the reserved Cashew Cream Sauce and carefully pour it over the broccoli and chicken. Toss gently to combine. Increase the heat to medium and continue to simmer, uncovered, for at least 5 minutes, or until the sauce has thickened slightly.

Just prior to serving, top everything with the flaxseed meal, if desired, to get that toasted bread crumb topping appearance, and serve directly from the skillet.

SPATCHCOCK CILANTRO LIME CHICKEN

Confession: Spatchcock was a totally new word to me last year, and I was a little intimidated by it. After I gave the method a try, it's now my preferred way to roast a whole chicken. By definition, spatchcock refers to removing the backbone in order to flatten the bird out for easy roasting. Since my family loves to eat easy roasted chicken (by far the most affordable way to buy it as well!), I spatchcock with the best of them at least once a month. This recipe is a zesty play on basic roast chicken for a simple dinner, or you can carve the meat, chop it and serve with your favorite salsa or guacamole recipes in lettuce cups for a creative spin on taco night!

Serves 4

---

1 whole organic, free-range chicken (about 4 pounds [1.8 kg])

Juice of 2 limes, about ⅓ cup (79 mL)

2 cloves garlic, well minced

1 tsp (5 g) coarse sea salt

½ tsp ground coriander

1 tbsp (15 g) coconut oil, melted

Additional squeeze of fresh lime juice

1 to 2 tbsp (5 g) chopped fresh cilantro

Preheat the oven to 425°F (218°C). Prepare the chicken by removing the innards, cleaning off any undesired bits from the skin and giving the whole thing a rinse under cold water. Pat dry.

Butterfly the chicken by removing the backbone with a large knife and, from the inside of the bird, cracking the breastbone just a bit so that the whole chicken lays flat when placed meat side up. The backbone can also be cut out with a sharp pair of kitchen shears. *Trust me, this is easier than it sounds.* Set the bird aside in a large resealable plastic bag and move on to the marinade.

In a small bowl, combine the lime juice, garlic, sea salt and coriander. Whisk in the melted coconut oil by slowly streaming it so that it emulsifies in the juice. Coconut oil melts at 76°F (24°C) and loves to solidify when mixed with other ingredients, so aggressively whisking helps to better incorporate it.

Pour the marinade over the chicken in the bag. With your hands on the outside of the bag, smooth the marinade into all the crevices, ensuring an even coat of flavor. Seal and set aside for 15 minutes.

Place the chicken breast side up on a rimmed baking sheet or a wide roasting pan with a flat roasting rack. Roast for 45 minutes, or until the internal temperature at the breast is 160°F (71°C). At the 35- to 40-minute mark, I like to baste the chicken in the run-off juices and coconut oil to help crisp the skin. That is optional, though.

When the chicken reaches 160°F (71°C), it can be removed from the oven. Be sure to cover the pan with foil and allow the bird to rest. Carryover cooking will jump the temperature up to a perfect 165°F to 170°F (74°C to 77°C) and the juices will redistribute back into the bird, giving you crispy skin on the outside and juicy meat on the inside.

Serve by giving the chicken a final squeeze of fresh lime juice and a sprinkling of chopped cilantro.

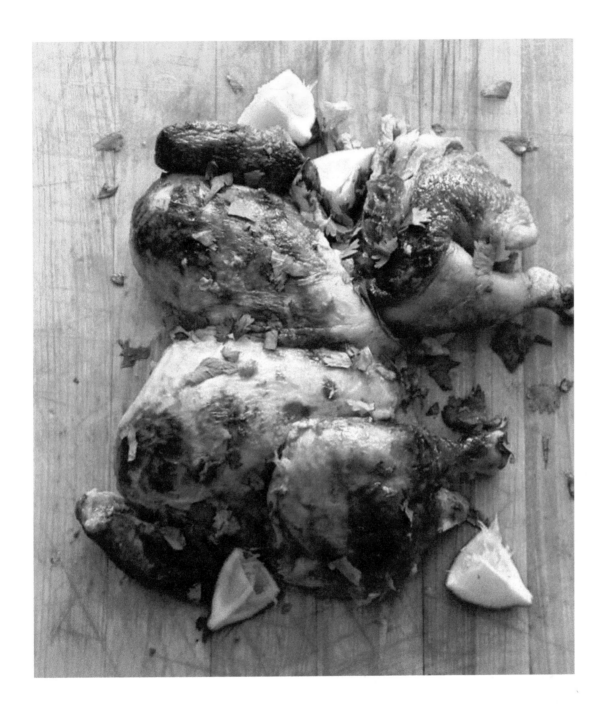

CHILI LIME TURKEY BURGERS

These turkey burgers steal the show thanks to spicy peppers, garlic and green onions. It's impressive how much flavor can be imparted into boring ground meat for less than the price of a latte.

Serves 4

---

1 lb (454 g) ground turkey

1 serrano (or jalapeño) pepper, seeded and finely diced

2 garlic cloves, minced

2 green onions, thinly sliced

Zest of half a lime

½ tsp kosher salt

1 egg

1 tbsp (15 g) coconut oil, if using an indoor grill or stovetop skillet

Sliced avocado or Spinach Guacamole Salsa (here), optional

Large lettuce leaves (optional)

Decide whether you intend to grill the burgers outdoors (or inside on an indoor grill) or if you'd rather cook them on the stovetop. Any option is fine, though I do like the flavor that comes from an outdoor grill. If using an outdoor grill, preheat it now.

To prepare the burgers, place the ground turkey in a large mixing bowl. Add the chile pepper, garlic, green onions, lime zest, kosher salt and egg.

Roll up your sleeves and use your hands to combine. It really is the best way to combine ingredients with ground meat. After the mixture is well mixed, divide it into four equal portions and shape into patties. Be sure to wash your hands well after this step (not that you would go about cooking with gooey meat hands … I hope).

If using an indoor grill or cooking these on the stovetop, preheat or turn the burner to medium-high and grease the indoor grill with some coconut oil (or melt the oil in a large skillet, if using the stovetop). Cook the burgers for about 5 minutes on each side. Ensure that the burgers are cooked through and no longer pink before serving (with an internal temperature of 165°F, which is 74°C) since poultry should not be undercooked.

Top with some avocado slices or even Spinach Guacamole Salsa (here) if you'd like, and wrap the burgers in large lettuce leaves.

ZESTY TURKEY MEATBALLS

Meatballs are one of those no-brainer standbys in Paleo. They are so versatile, inexpensive and easy to prepare. In fact, once you find a method you like, it's very easy to adapt recipes to your liking. For this one, I'm using lean ground turkey with zesty Fajita Seasoning Blend. Refer to my list of 15 Salt-Free, 5-Ingredient-or-Less Seasoning Blends (here-190) for other tasty ideas to experiment with in place of the smoky, spicy fajita blend. I'm sure you'll come up with something great!

Serves 3 to 4

1 pound (454 g) ground turkey

1 egg

1 batch Fajita Seasoning Blend

(here)

1 tsp (5 g) kosher salt

1 tsp (5 g) garlic powder

¼ cup (28 g) coconut flour

Preheat the oven to 400°F (204°C). Select a baking sheet or pan for baking the meatballs. Because these meatballs are virtually fat free, be sure to use a nonstick surface such as parchment paper or a silicone mat if you don't have a nonstick roasting pan.

In a mixing bowl, thoroughly combine all of the ingredients by hand before shaping into balls. When it comes to incorporating ingredients into ground meat, there simply is no better tool than your hands. Be sure to wash up after handling raw meat.

Use that quarter measuring cup as a scoop, so that each meatball is uniform. Scoop the meatball mixture out with the cup (or something comparable—the goal here is consistency) and shape into a ball using the palms of your hands. Arrange the meatballs on the baking sheet evenly spaced from each other. There should be a dozen.

Bake for about 25 to 30 minutes, or until the internal temperature of a meatball reaches between 160°F (71°C) and 170°F (77°C). Because it's poultry, the outside won't reach a deep brown, so be cautious not to overcook the meatballs in pursuit of that familiar golden crust.

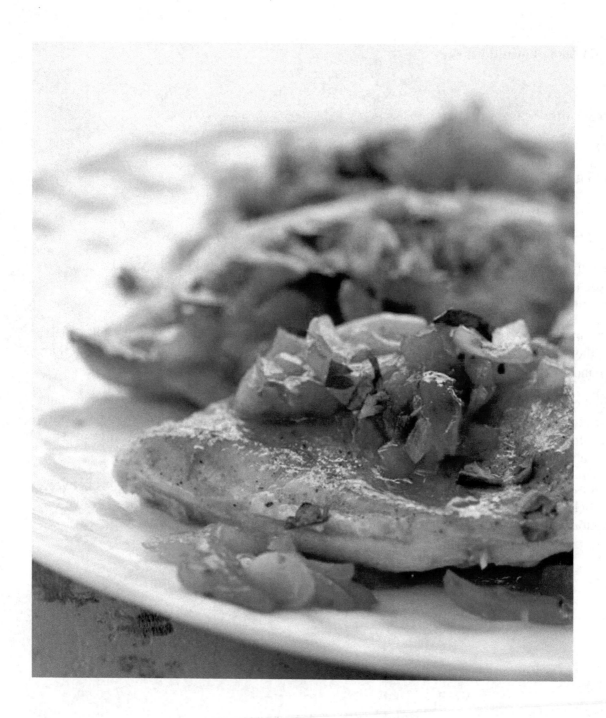

TUESDAY NIGHT CHICKEN

Truthfully, this could be named after any day of the week. It's so approachable and affordable that you won't hesitate to make it after a long day at work or just before payday hits. This recipe highlights my favorite way to cook a rich tomato sauce quickly: red-pepper flakes and cinnamon. It's how my Italian grandmother fed our family, so naturally I consider it the right way, as any true Italian would. Enjoy using these straightforward ingredients to create a bold and flavorful classic Italian dinner … any night of the week.

Serves 2 to 4

2 large boneless, skinless chicken breasts (about 1 pound [454 g])

1 tsp (5 g) House Seasoning Blend (here)

Extra virgin olive oil

1 cup (150 g) diced white or yellow onion

2 cloves garlic, minced

1 batch Italian Seasoning Blend (here)

½ tsp kosher salt

¼ tsp ground cinnamon

1 (14.5 oz [411 g]) can fire-roasted tomatoes

Fresh basil and/or flat-leaf parsley, for garnish

Prepare the chicken breasts first by filleting lengthwise to make 2 thick breasts into 4 thinner ones. Dust both sides with the House Seasoning Blend.

Heat a high-sided skillet over medium-high heat and add a little bit of olive oil to the pan—enough just to coat the bottom. When the oil is hot, lay the seasoned chicken breasts in to sear. Work in batches to avoid overcrowding the pan as overcrowding leads to steaming, not browning. When the chicken has been seared (note, not fully cooked) on both sides, transfer it to a plate and set aside.

Reduce the temperature to medium and replenish the pan with a little more olive oil if it looks dry. Add the onion, garlic, Italian Seasoning Blend, kosher salt and cinnamon and cook, stirring often. If you are not accustomed to building sauces this way, I know it may appear a bit strange, but trust me on this. Applying heat and oil to the dried herbs prior to immersing them in liquid revives the oils and creates a deeper flavor. It's the trick to crafting a rich tomato sauce in such a short amount of time.

Cook until the onion is translucent and the garlic and herbs fragrant. Pour in the fire-roasted tomatoes and mix together. When the sauce bubbles, add the par-cooked chicken back to the pan, nestle it into the spiced-tomato-goodness, cover and reduce the temperature to a simmer.

Simmer for 15 to 20 minutes while chopping the fresh garnishes—use either or both basil or flat-leaf parsley. This final simmer also allows plenty of time to whip up a quick vegetable side like an easy salad, sautéed dark leafy greens or Pan-Roasted Cauliflower and Zucchini (here).

I like to serve this directly from the pan after scattering it with the vibrant green fresh herbs.

EASY THAI COCONUT CHICKEN

This recipe transforms basic chicken and vegetables into something exotic and fantastic thanks to a couple of dynamic, yet accessible, ingredients: coconut milk and green curry paste. These ingredients can be found in any grocery store; no additional stops at expensive health stores required.

Serves 4

---

1 (13.6 oz [403 mL]) can full-fat organic coconut milk

1 tbsp (45 mL) green curry paste

1 tbsp (45 g) coconut oil

1 pound (454 g) boneless, skinless chicken breasts (see note)

½ tsp plus a pinch kosher salt

½ cup (75 g) sliced carrots (cut into coins)

1 cup (150 g) diced onion

2 cloves garlic, minced

1 cup (150 g) sliced zucchini (cut into half-moon shapes)

½ cup (40 g) sliced white mushrooms

1 tbsp (45 g) seeded and sliced fresh red chile pepper

In a small bowl, combine the coconut milk with the green curry paste. Set aside.

Preheat a large, high-sided skillet with a lid over medium-high heat and melt the coconut oil in the pan.

Meanwhile, cut the chicken breasts into 2-inch (5-cm) cubes and season one side with a sprinkling of kosher salt.

When the coconut oil is hot, drop the cubed chicken into the pan. This is one time when you don't want to stir the meat while it cooks. Let the chicken sear, undisturbed, for about 5 minutes before turning the cubes to a second side to sear for about 3 minutes.

Reduce the heat to medium, then add the carrots, onion and garlic to the chicken. Cook and stir for about 4 minutes. Add the zucchini, mushrooms, chile pepper slices and the remaining ½ teaspoon salt.

Continue to cook and stir for another 5 minutes. If at any point the pan is getting too dark with what looks like burnt bits on the bottom, use about ¼ cup (60 mL) of water to deglaze the pan. Deglazing means that liquid is used to loosen the browned bits stuck to the bottom of a hot pan during the cooking process. The liquid "lifts" them up and incorporates the browned bits as added flavor to the dish. If you need to do that while you prepare this portion of the recipe, do it. If the browned bits are not overwhelming the pan, don't worry about it.

When the zucchini and mushrooms are golden brown, pour in the coconut milk mixture. Simmer for 8 to 10 minutes to reduce the coconut milk slightly and concentrate the flavors.

I recommend serving this dish over cauliflower rice (see here) or eating it as a chunky soup, garnished with fresh basil—regular, sweet or Thai basil is fine.

For a pescatarian variation, 1 pound of prawns (about 31 to 40 per pound [1 kg] size is ideal) can be substituted. Select wild prawns that have been shelled and deveined, for added convenience. Cook the vegetables as directed, then add the prawns to the pan at the same time as the coconut milk mixture. The prawns will cook as the coconut milk simmers and thickens.

Note: Prawns can be substituted for chicken for a seafood option, or double the recipe and use both chicken and prawns to feed a crowd!

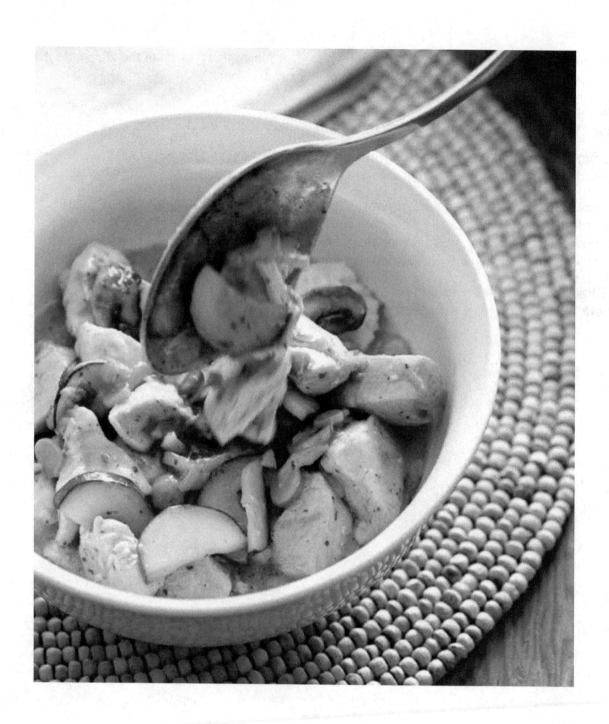

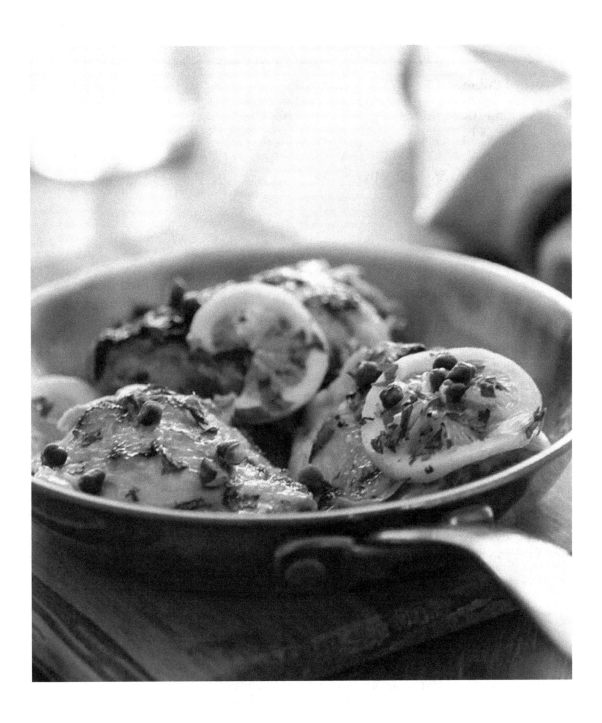

CRISPY CHICKEN WITH LEMON AND CAPERS

Few items are as affordable as bone-in, skin-on chicken thighs, and this is one of my favorite ways to make them. It seems like I always have parsley and a lemon hanging around my kitchen, and I generally pre-make a batch of House Seasoning Blend, since I use it on almost everything. This dish takes just over 30 minutes to throw together and finishes in the oven, leaving plenty of time to whip up a quick vegetable side dish and tidy up the kitchen. As a busy mom, I rely on meals like this one.

Serves 2 to 4

2 lb (908 g) chicken thighs

1 tsp House Seasoning Blend (here)

½ tsp kosher salt

2 to 3 tbsp (30 to 45 mL) extra virgin olive oil

1 tsp (5 g) capers

1 tbsp (3 g) chopped fresh flat-leaf parsley

1 lemon, sliced

Preheat the oven to 375°F (190°C). Trim any excess fat or hanging skin away from the thighs. Season the skin side of the thighs with the House Seasoning Blend and kosher salt and set aside.

Heat a cast-iron skillet (or another oven-safe pan) to medium-high and add the olive oil. If there won't be about an inch or so (3 cm) of space in between each thigh once arranged in the pan, work in batches instead. Attempting to do them all at once in a pan that is too small will cause the temperature of the pan to drop quickly, steaming the thighs rather than searing them.

Sear the chicken skin side down for 2 to 3 minutes, then set the first round aside while the second batch sears. Return all of the chicken to the skillet skin side up and transfer the skillet to the oven. Roast for 30 minutes.

Remove the skillet from the oven and sprinkle the chicken with the capers and parsley. Squeeze the juice of the lemon over the top of the chicken while it's still in the skillet. Arranged the squeezed lemon slices in the skillet with the chicken and serve directly from the pan. Be sure to spoon plenty of the pan juices over the chicken when serving; it's delicious.

CHICKEN AND CHORIZO STEW

This soup filled my Dutch oven to the brim and cost me next to nothing to make. Can you believe I fed 6 hungry adults for less than twenty bucks? This stew starts with basic meat and potatoes then adds fresh tomatoes and lots of spice. Thanks to a well-stocked spice cupboard, it was just a pinch of this and a dash of that and voilà! Soup's on!

Serves 6 to 8

1 tbsp (15 g) lard, tallow or duck fat (preferred)

3 cups (475 g) diced white or yellow onions

4 cloves garlic, minced

12 oz to 16 oz (340 g to 454 g) fresh pork chorizo sausage

4 cups (600 g) diced white sweet potatoes

4 cups (about 2 lb [908 g]) diced tomatoes

1 tbsp (15 g) Adobo Seasoning Blend (here)

2 tsp (10 g) coarse sea salt

½ tsp red-pepper flakes

5 cups (1.2 L) chicken stock

1 lb (454 g) boneless, skinless chicken breasts

Toppings: thinly sliced radishes, sliced avocado, lime wedges and fresh cilantro. Fresh jalapeño slices are welcome for those looking for some extra heat.

Heat a Dutch oven or another large stockpot with a lid over medium heat and melt the fat. (I prefer lard in this recipe.)

Add the onions, garlic and chorizo and cook until the onions have softened, about 6 to 7 minutes. Then add the sweet potatoes, tomatoes, adobo seasoning, sea salt and pepper flakes and stir to combine. Now pour in the chicken stock and bring to a boil.

Once the broth is bubbling, carefully lower in the whole chicken breasts. They will poach in the spicy broth over the next hour.

Cover the pot and reduce the temperature to a simmer. Let the soup bubble away. Meanwhile, prepare the fresh toppings and store in the refrigerator until it's time to eat.

After an hour or so, remove the chicken and shred. Add it back to the pot and stir everything together once more. It's done!

To serve, ladle portions into individual bowls and layer in the fresh avocado slices, a small handful of thinly sliced radishes, freshly torn cilantro and a squeeze from a lime wedge. If you'd like extra heat, why not throw a few jalapeño slices on top as well? Serve the stew right away.

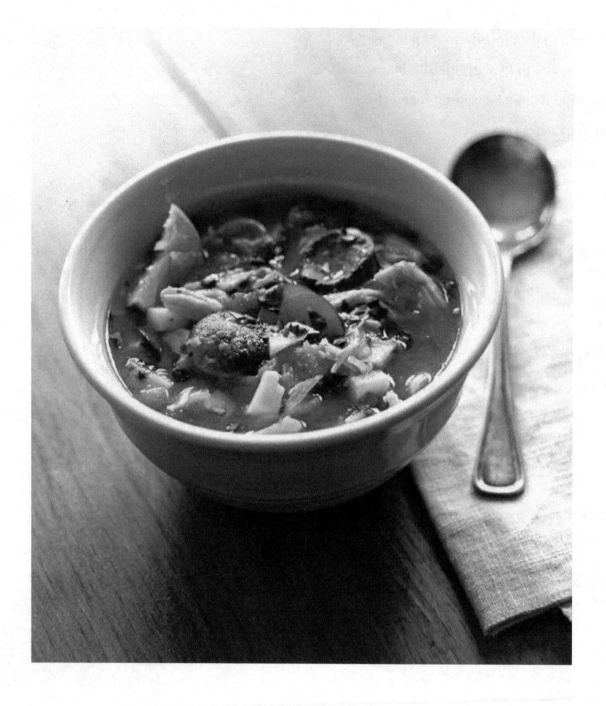

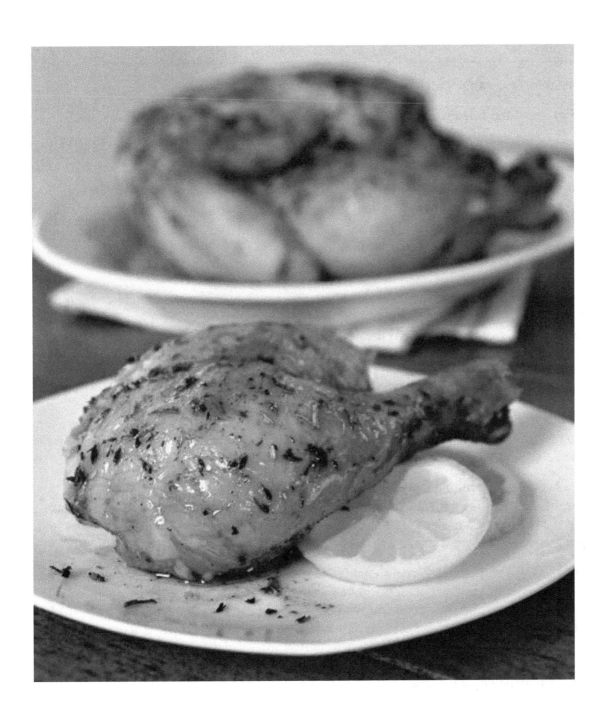

ROASTED FRENCH COUNTRYSIDE CHICKEN

Herbs, lemon and grass-fed butter smothered over the perfect roasted chicken. Does dinner get any better? Spend the extra bucks on a quality organic, free-range chicken. Buy one that was able to eat bugs—not soy, corn or whatever else is put into vegetarian feed these days. Chickens are not vegetarians! Buy a chicken that lived a happy life and prepare it with these simple ingredients for a fine family meal that prioritizes quality, for them and for us.

Serves 4

1 whole organic, free-range chicken (about 4 pounds [1.8 kg])

3 tbsp (45 g) grass-fed butter, at room temperature

1 batch French Countryside Seasoning Blend (here)

½ tsp coarse sea salt

¼ tsp fresh cracked black pepper

1 lemon

Preheat the oven to 400°F (204°C).

Remove the innards from the chicken and rinse both the inside and outside of the bird. Trim the tail off and any excess skin and fat at the bottom opening. Use a sharp knife or a pair of kitchen shears to remove the exposed portion of the neck (if it is still intact) by cutting along both sides of the spine, about an inch (2.5 cm) or so, then pull back the neck and cut across, severing it from the backbone. (This is what real, whole foods cooking looks like, folks.) Pat dry with a disposable towel—really get the bird dry so the skin crisps well. Set it aside.

The key to this roasted chicken is the herbed compound butter. Take your room temperature, grass-fed butter and combine it with the French Countryside Seasoning Blend, sea salt and black pepper. I use a regular spoon to mix this up, plus it comes in handy for the next step.

Return the chicken to the cutting board and lay breast side up. Next, make a pocket to access the meat under the skin. Lift the skin at the base of the chicken and, using a sharp paring knife, cut the silky tissue between the breast meat and the skin. Also trim into the leg sockets to expose the thigh and leg meat as best you can.

Use the spoon to usher in bits of the compound butter. Guide the spoonfuls of flavorful butter into the pocket under the skin and then from the outside push against the spoon to slide the butter off. Then manipulate it from the outside, moving the herbed butter evenly over the breast, thigh and leg meat. Do this to both sides (left and right), reserving a little bit of butter for the exterior skin. And if a spoon's not working for you, just get your fingers in there and distribute the butter. Picture the flavor that you're imparting into the meat by this method; it helps you get through this step if it's making you a bit squeamish.

Rub the last of the compound butter on the skin of the bird. Hands make the best tool to get this job done. Place the bird on a roasting rack or in a roasting pan breast side up, then get your hands washed up.

Slice the lemon in half and squeeze the juice from half of it onto the skin, then stick both sections into the cavity of the bird to act as an aromatic while it roasts. Sprinkle on a pinch of sea salt and crack some fresh black pepper over the breast. Use butcher twine to truss (or "tie up") the drumsticks, and it's ready to roast.

Roast the chicken for 30 minutes, then reduce the oven temperature to 375°F (190°C) and roast for 1 hour. The meat is done when the internal temperature of the breast meat is at 165°F (74°C).

Before carving the chicken, allow it to rest out of the oven for 10 minutes so the juices redistribute into the meat.

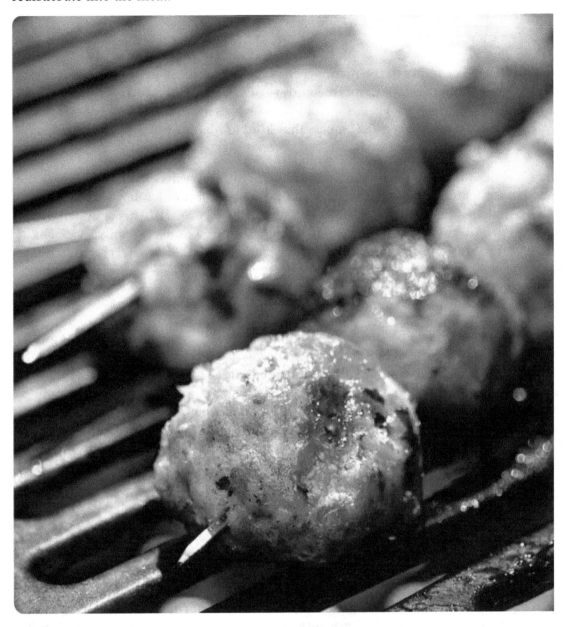

The first thing to know about pork is that quality is essential. Because pork is a fattier protein in general than, say, chicken, seafood or eggs, there is an increased risk of consuming harmful toxins if eating anything other than pasture-raised, organic pork. Since toxins are stored in fat and not in the liver as many mistakenly presume, it is critical to be a picky Paleo pork purveyor.

Use www.eatwild.com to find a farmer near you who is putting in the extra effort to raise pigs right, and get on his or her list for a whole or half hog each year. Stock your freezer full of delicious shoulders and loin, ribs and bellies for a fraction of what you'd pay for it wrapped under cellophane. If buying in bulk isn't an option, make a compromise by prioritizing pasture-raised pork for fattier cuts and then save a few bucks on a leaner one like tenderloin.

On bacon …

Bacon is no doubt a silver lining to the dietary restrictions that come with Paleo. As long as it's sourced from pastured pigs, is nitrite free and wasn't cured with added flavor enhancers like sugar, MSG or gluten-based colorings or preservatives, bacon is perfectly acceptable. However, finding bacon that meets that kind of quality usually comes with a steep price tag. So what's a person to do?

Enter Ciarra's Rules for Common Sense Eating: if an item is expensive, do not use it as the primary protein for a meal. Instead of relying on bacon or premium tenderloin for weekly meal rotations, make Ginger Peach Pulled Pork (here), Pork Tacos 101 (here) or Tangy Apricot Pulled Pork (here) —recipes that yield enough to feed a hungry family twice. Or take advantage of a sale on ground pork by making some Aloha Sliders (here) with fresh pineapple relish or a batch of Pot Sticker Meatballs (here). I'm a fan of eating; I'm not a fan of being strapped for cash at the end of every month. These recipes are the backbone of dinner planning, keeping our tummies full and our budget in check.

But back to bacon. In my home we do eat it—regularly, in fact. I generally have a pound or so in the house each week. Now, if breakfast for four was 2 pounds (900 g) of bacon, plus 8 scrambled eggs, a pint of fresh organic berries and a couple of avocados every day, we'd go broke. Therefore, I next to never serve bacon this way. Instead, I stretch the purchase by using it strategically in recipes where it is not the main ingredient. Crumble bacon bits into veggie scrambles with breakfast rather than serving slices on the side, or wrap it around veggies for an appetizer or lunch such as with Balsamic Bacon Brussels Bites (here).

The take-away here is that where a larger shoulder may be a staple for protein, bacon is not. Forgive the metaphor, but think of it this way: Shoulder is the cake, bacon is the frosting.

TEQUILA CARNITAS

Carnitas are my very favorite thing to eat since going Paleo. Affordable pork shoulder simply seasoned and slowly braised gets my vote every time. But all of that aside, let's talk about the elephant in the room: Is tequila Paleo? The short answer is yes. Any variety other than "Joven" or gold tequila will do, since that particular one is flavored with caramel coloring and is likely not gluten-free. Otherwise, *"resposado"* and *"anejo"* tequila comes from a plant, is gluten-free and contains no added sugars or artificial ingredients. That, my friends, gets tequila on the Paleo-friendly ingredient list and therefore into my Dutch oven with a hunk of pork and a twist of lime. Pile this on top of a batch of cauliflower rice or a baked sweet potato and you've got a meal deserving of a social media share!

Serves 6 to 8

3 lb (1.3 kg) boneless pork shoulder

1 batch Taco Seasoning Blend (here)

1 tsp (5 g) kosher salt

2 to 3 tbsp (30 to 45 g) lard or coconut oil

1 small onion, thinly sliced

5 cloves garlic, crushed

1 large jalapeño, seeded and fined minced (about ¼ cup [45 g])

Juice of 2 limes, about ½ cup (118 mL)

1 cup (237 mL) pure tequila (gluten-free, no added sugars)

½ cup (118 mL) water

Fresh cilantro and additional lime wedges, for garnish

Cut the pork shoulder into four or five even chunks and coat with the Taco Seasoning Blend, plus the kosher salt.

Heat a Dutch oven over medium-high heat and melt the lard or coconut oil (though lard is my favorite). Drop in the seasoned pork and sear the sides. If the spices are starting to burn, reduce the temperature just a bit. It's also a good idea to work in batches to avoid overcrowding the pan. If too many chunks of meat go in together, the result will be steaming, not searing. Not pretty.

Once seared, return all of the meat to the pan and drop in the onion, garlic and jalapeño. Lightly mix the ingredients, but make sure the pork gets priority at the bottom of the dog-pile.

Next, pour in the fresh lime juice, tequila and water. Bring to a boil, then reduce the temperature to a simmer and cover.

Let the pork braise on the stovetop for 2 hours, or until it falls apart easily when gently pressed with the back of a fork.

Remove the Dutch oven from the heat, shred the pork (discard any fatty bits) and mix with the juices. Scoop all the pork out, transfer to a baking dish and pop it under the broiler for a few minutes to crisp up the carnitas. Just eyeball it.

Pour the remaining braising liquid over the carnitas and serve with fresh cilantro and a few lime wedges for squeezing. Other toppings that go great with carnitas are avocado, sliced radishes, finely diced red onion and even fresh pineapple, if you're feeling adventurous.

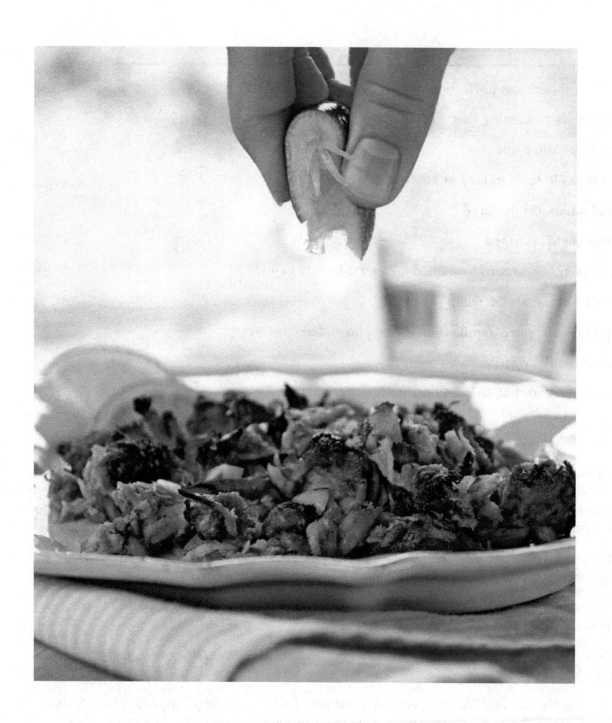

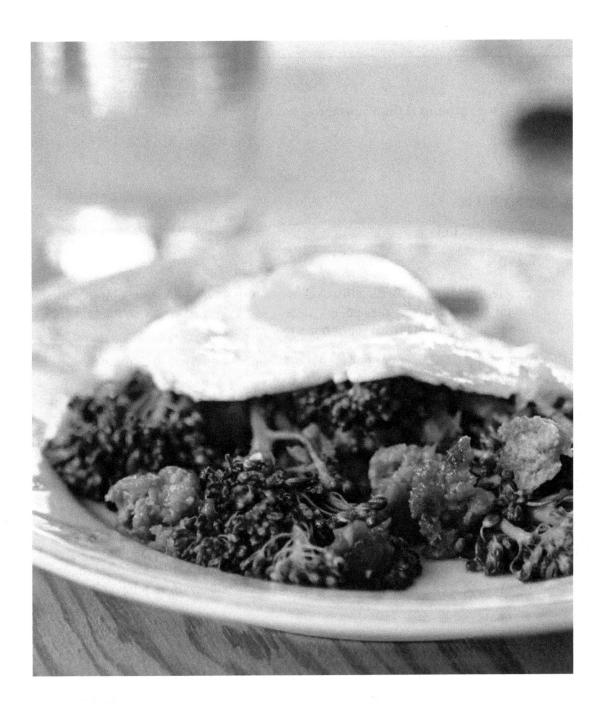

SAUSAGE AND BROCCOLINI

Whether it's a hearty breakfast or easy dinner you're after, Sausage and Broccolini will hit the spot. Every Paleo purveyor has a few recipes in their back pocket for those days when we don't feel like spending an hour in the kitchen, and this is one of mine. The whole family eats for less than a drive-thru fast-food run or gluten-free pizza delivery.

Can't find Broccolini? Regular broccoli makes a fine substitute. Be sure to cut the florets in half to keep the cooking time consistent.

Serves 2 to 4

Extra virgin olive oil

12 to 16 oz (340 to 454 g) ground Italian sausage

1 clove garlic, minced

¼ tsp kosher salt

Pinch of red-pepper flakes

1 lb (454 g) organic Broccolini

2 to 4 eggs (optional)

Start by preheating a large skillet, one with a lid, over medium-high heat. Drizzle a bit of extra virgin olive oil into the pan to help the sausage get started. Just eyeball this. When the oil is hot, crumble in the sausage and begin to brown for about 5 to 7 minutes.

Add the garlic, kosher salt and red-pepper flakes to the sausage. Cook for 2 to 3 minutes and stir until the sausage is nearly done. Some brown bits will coat the bottom of the pan, which may make it look like it's burning, but it's so not—that browning is great flavor waiting to be lifted back into the meat!

Trim the Broccolini to remove any dried ends from the stalks. Place the Broccolini on top of the browned sausage; do not mix! Instead, reduce the temperature to low and cover the pan with a secure lid. After 8 to 10 minutes, remove the lid and toss the Broccolini and sausage together. Notice how the steam from the Broccolini deglazed the pan and loosened those brown bits? That's exactly what we want. Combine and serve hot.

This is excellent with a runny fried egg on top! If you'd like to eat it with an egg on top, fry a few to your preference while the Broccolini is steaming so both are ready for serving at the same time. A runny yolk over par-cooked Broccolini and spicy Italian sausage is unbelievably delicious!

CAULIFLOWER LASAGNA

There are many grain-free pasta substitutions out there made from nuts, coconut and other fancier ingredients. However, one day I thought, "Why not give cauliflower a shot?" It totally worked. This lasagna has become a fan-favorite for the past year on Popular Paleo. Hit up your local wholesale retailer for great deals on bulk organic vegetables and get this nutritious grain-free, dairy-free lasagna in your oven tonight!

Serves 6 to 8

FOR THE LASAGNA NOODLES

1 head cauliflower (6 cups [1.9 kg]), chopped

2 to 3 cloves garlic

½ tsp kosher salt

1 tsp (3 g) dried Italian seasoning

2 eggs

FOR THE BOLOGNESE

2 tbsp (30 mL) extra virgin olive oil

2 to 3 carrots, chopped (1 cup [150 g])

1 small onion, diced

1 rib celery, diced

1 tsp (5 g) kosher salt

1 tsp (3 g) dried basil

1 tsp (3 g) dried oregano

⅛ tsp cinnamon (and barely ⅛ tsp … it's a dusting of cinnamon!)

Pinch of red-pepper flakes (less than 10 flakes)

3 cloves garlic, minced

12 oz (340 g) ground Italian sausage

1 (14.5 oz [411 g]) can organic diced tomatoes

1 (15 oz [425 g]) can organic tomato sauce

1 cup (237 mL) organic chicken stock

A couple handfuls of baby spinach and chopped fresh basil (optional)

Start by making the cauliflower noodles. Preheat the oven to 350°F (177°C). Remove the leaves and core from the head of cauliflower and chop the cauliflower into very small pieces. I use my knife, but you can certainly do this in a food processor.

Steam the cauliflower until fully cooked but not mushy, about 6 minutes. While the cauliflower still hot, use a potato masher or pastry cutter to break down the cauliflower. Cauliflower releases a fair amount of liquid while it cooks, so drain as much liquid from the cauliflower as possible. Use cheesecloth or a bag used for making nut milks, or even just press against the cooked cauliflower with the back of a wooden spoon to release the excess liquid.

Once cauliflower has been drained, add the garlic, kosher salt and Italian seasoning and combine. Last, add the eggs to the mixture and transfer to a baking sheet lined with a silicone mat or parchment paper. Since there is no fat in this cauliflower "noodle," it will stick to an unlined baking sheet.

Depending on which casserole or lasagna pan you plan to use, spread the cauliflower "noodle" out to a size that will provide enough for 2 layers once assembled. For example, the casserole dish I use is your basic oval 2.8 liter baker (8 inch by 11 inch by 3 inch [20 cm by 28 cm by 8 cm]), so I spread my cauliflower out a half inch (one centimeter) thick on a standard American 17 inch by 12 inch (43 cm by 31 cm) baking sheet. Spreading the cauliflower out to this size will allow me to cut it in half and have 2 cauliflower "noodles" to layer in my lasagna pan.

Bake for 45 minutes. It needs to be a little overcooked and dried out since it will soon be layered with a bolognese.

While the cauliflower bakes, make the bolognese.

Classic bolognese starts with mirepoix (carrot, onion and celery), and that's what we're going to do here. Heat a large skillet with high sides (or a Dutch oven) over medium-high heat. Drizzle in the olive oil.

While the oil comes to temp, add the carrots, onion and celery. Sprinkle with the kosher salt and other seasonings. It will look a bit strange if you're not in the habit of building sauces in this order, but roll with it. This method gets the oils going and rehydrates the dried herbs before the tomatoes hit. Cook and stir frequently for about 4 to 5 minutes, then add the garlic and the sausage.

Cook until the sausage has browned, about 6 to 8 minutes. Add the diced tomatoes, tomato sauce and chicken stock to the pot. Reduce the heat to medium low and stir and simmer for about 15 minutes. Cover if your sauce starts to dry out (or if it's splattering everywhere and making a mess of your stove).

When the cauliflower "noodle" has finished cooking, remove it from the oven and transfer to a large cutting board or work surface. Depending on the size and shape of your lasagna pan (and thus the size and shape of your cauli-noodle), divide into 2 sections that will perfectly layer your lasagna. Remove the bolognese from the heat and grab your baking dish.

BUILD THE LASAGNA BY LAYERING:

1. about a cup (237 mL) of sauce

2. a cauliflower "noodle"

3. half of the remaining sauce

4. a couple handfuls of baby spinach, if using

5. the second cauliflower "noodle"

6. the remaining sauce

Cover and bake at 350°F (177°C) for about 20 to 25 minutes—just enough to bring everything together and for the sauce to bubble around the edges.

Garnish with fresh basil for a dairy-free, grain-free delicious lasagna!

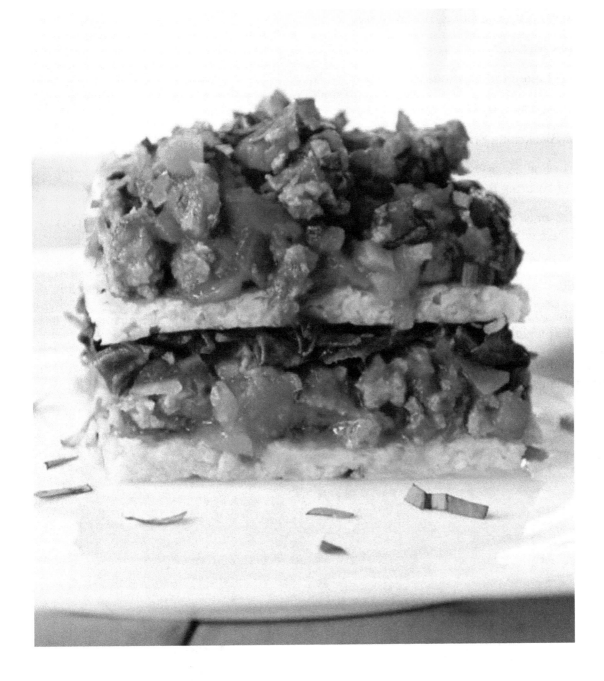

OVEN-BLACKENED PULLED PORK

Did I have you at oven? No need to fuss over an outdoor grill or smoker. This convenient recipe is my go-to for both a crowd pleaser and batch-cooking day alike. Picking up a bone-in shoulder of pork always equals savings at the register, and the Blackening Seasoning Blend couldn't be simpler. Just season the pork, pop it in the oven and hours later you have pulled pork that's a little too good for the amount of effort and expense on your part.

Serves 4 to 6

1 batch Blackening Seasoning Blend (here)

1 tsp (5 g) kosher salt

3 lb (1.4 kg) bone-in pork shoulder

Preheat the oven to 300°F (149°C).

Prepare the Blackening Seasoning Blend from here, plus add in the kosher salt.

Pat the pork shoulder dry with a paper towel and rub with the seasoning blend, evenly coating the pork and ensuring the seasonings are rubbed into any crevices.

Place the seasoned pork into a large roasting pan and pop in the oven for 5 hours (uncovered). Most shoulders will have a side that is predominantly fat; be sure to have that side facing up.

The pork is done when the meat falls apart easily with just gentle pressure from the back of a fork. Be sure it has reached an internal temperature of at least 150°F (66°C) as well to be safe.

Let it rest for 10 minutes after removing from the oven, then pull the pork apart one meaty section at a time. Discard any large pieces of fat or repurpose, if you choose.

Serve the pulled pork as is or as the star of any number of delicious recipes, such as pork stuffed peppers, frittatas or piled high on baked sweet potatoes.

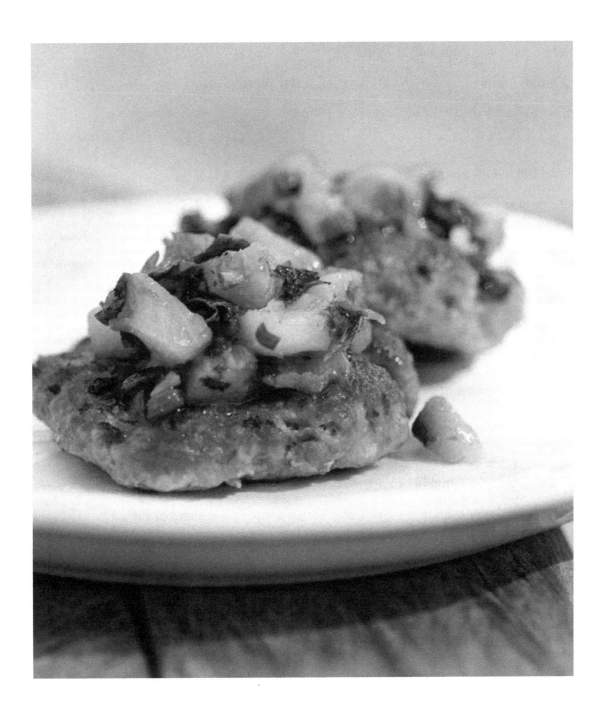

ALOHA SLIDERS WITH PINEAPPLE RELISH

The secret's in the sauce—or so they say. And this sauce—well, relish—is fresh, spicy, sweet and just plain delicious. It's the perfect accompaniment to savory grilled pork sliders. This recipe "wows" without breaking the bank!

Serves 4 to 6

FOR THE RELISH

2 tbsp (30 g) unrefined coconut oil

1 small red onion (about 2 inches [5 cm] across), finely diced

1 jalapeño, seeded and finely diced Zest from 1 lime

¼ tsp sea salt

2 to 2 ½ cups (400 to 600 g) diced pineapple (see note)

¼ cup (10 g) chopped cilantro

FOR THE SLIDERS

1 ½ to 2 lb (683 to 908 g) ground pork

1 clove garlic, minced

¼ cup (10 g) chopped cilantro

¼ cup (40 g) finely diced red onion

½ tsp ground cumin

½ tsp kosher salt

To start the relish, heat a large pan over medium heat and melt the coconut oil. Once the oil is hot (is glossy and slides easily from side to side when tilted), add the onion, jalapeño, lime zest and sea salt. Cook until the onion is just about translucent, about 10 minutes.

Add the pineapple and mix everything together. Because pineapple contains a fair amount of natural sugar, it's important that the pan temperature stays around medium. Any hotter and the sugars will burn before the pineapple has enough time to soften. Also, pineapple that's cooked too quickly won't release the sugary juices that create the spicy glaze we need for the sliders. So take your time, keep the temperature moderate and gently stir frequently. The sauce will take about 25 to 30 minutes to finish. It's done when the pineapple has a nice caramel color to it and is slightly softened, but not mushy.

Remove it from the heat, mix in the chopped cilantro and cover until the sliders are ready to be sauced.

While the sauce simmers, in a large bowl, combine the ingredients for the sliders by hand. There really is no better way to combine ingredients into ground meat than by hand.

When the ingredients are evenly distributed in the ground pork, shape into 6 even patties.

Heat the grill to medium high, or about 400°F (204°C), and place the sliders on the grate. Grill undisturbed for 5 to 6 minutes, then turn and grill the other side for 4 to 6 minutes. The cue to know whether or not the sliders are ready to be turned (or are done) is when the meat easily lifts away from the grate. Meat will naturally release when grilling, making it easy to know when the time is right to turn it or remove it.

When the sliders are no longer pink and have an internal temperature of 160°F (71°C), remove them from the grill and place on a serving dish or individual plates. Give the spicy pineapple relish a stir, then spoon the desired amount over the tops of the sliders and serve hot.

Note: There is some flexibility when it comes to the pineapple, since it's not always affordable when out of season. Use either fresh pineapple that's been peeled, cored and cubed into bite-size pieces or 1 (20 oz [567 g]) can pineapple chunks or 2 (8 oz [225 g]) cans pineapple chunks. If using canned pineapple, be sure to drain the juice before adding to the pan. Do not use crushed pineapple.

SZECHWAN PEASANT PORK

This is part ribs, part spicy broth–kind of like soup with a hunk of pork in it. The thing I love about "peasant" recipes is that they're good because they have to be. These dishes cannot hide behind impressive gourmet ingredients. Rich flavors from inexpensive ingredients are lured out by tried-and-true preparation methods. The Chinese have this in the bag, if you ask me.

My advice for attacking this spicy dish is to alternate nibbling on the pork sparerib with a hefty spoonful of spicy broth, onion and peppers. Enjoy this with sweet potato, kelp or shirataki noodles or even some cauliflower rice for a fine Chinese-inspired meal.

Serves 4 to 6

---

3 lb (1.4 kg) bone-in pork spareribs

1 tsp (5 g) kosher salt

2 tbsp (30 g) Paleo-friendly fat (animal-based fats work better in this dish)

1 large white or yellow onion, cut into ⅛-inch-thick (3-mm-thick) slices

8 red chilies, whole

10 cloves garlic, crushed

1 tsp (5 g) Korean hot pepper powder (crushed red-pepper flakes can be substituted)

4 cups (948 mL) chicken stock (homemade is best)

1 cup (237 mL) coconut aminos

Chopped fresh cilantro and sliced green onions

Slice the rack of spareribs into singles or ask your butcher to do it for you. Generously season the meaty portions of the ribs with the kosher salt.

Heat a Dutch oven or large heavy-bottomed pot with a secure-fitting lid over medium-high heat and melt your choice of Paleo-friendly fat. Flavor-wise, I prefer to use an animal-based fat like lard, tallow or duck fat. However, coconut or avocado oil will work as well.

When the fat is hot (glossy and moves easily across the pan when tilted from side to side), sear the salted spareribs. Arrange the ribs meat side down, being careful not to overcrowd the pan. Work in batches if necessary. Placing the ribs too close to each other will drop the temperature of the pan, resulting in the ribs being steamed.

After the spareribs are seared, return all of the meat to the Dutch oven and top with the onion, whole red chili peppers, garlic and Korean hot pepper powder (or red-pepper flakes). Pour the stock and coconut aminos over the meat and veggies and bring to a boil. (Leave the temperature at medium high.)

When the stock boils, cover the Dutch oven and reduce the temperature to low. Ideally, the stock should bubble a bit, but not reach a rolling boil during the braising time.

Braise, covered, for about 3 hours, then remove the lid and let the mixture simmer uncovered to reduce the liquid by 25 percent or so and concentrate the flavors. When the braising liquid has gone down enough that the tops of the ribs are visible (after about 20 minutes), skim off as much of the fat layer from the top of the broth as you're able. Discard the skimmed fat.

The pork is ready to serve! I like to present this family style, topped with chopped cilantro and sliced green onions.

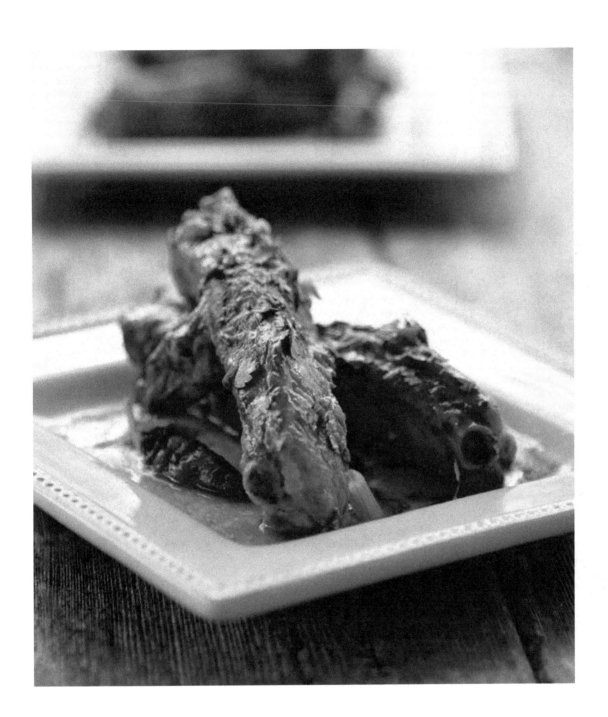

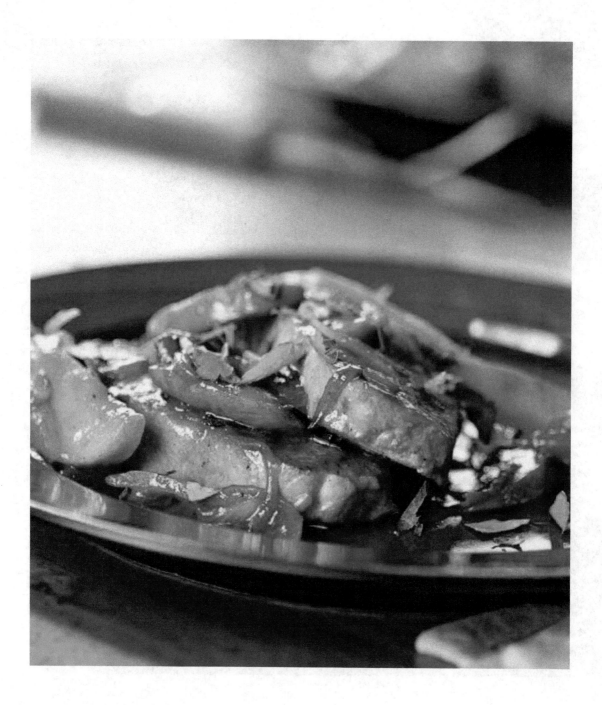

PALEO PORK NORMANDY

Pork Normandy highlights lean pork loin chops with the sweet and savory flavors of apple and onion, brought together with a tangy sauce from reduced hard apple cider. There are a handful of variations out there, but this one keeps it Paleo and is affordable enough to make any night of the week.

Serves 4

4 boneless pork loin chops

Coarse sea salt, to taste, plus 1 tsp (5 g)

Black pepper, to taste

2 tbsp (30 g) grass-fed butter or ghee, divided

½ large white or yellow onion, sliced

⅛-inch (3-mm) thick

1 large sweet apple, such as Honeycrisp

1 bay leaf

½ tsp dried thyme (or 1 tsp [3 g] fresh thyme)

1 cup (237 mL) hard apple cider (Be sure it is gluten-free without added sugar.)

Chopped fresh Italian flat-leaf parsley, for garnish (optional)

Trim excess fat from the outsides of the pork loin chops and season liberally with sea salt and black pepper.

Heat a large skillet over medium-high heat and drop in 1 tablespoon (15 g) of the butter or ghee. Sear both sides of the pork, about 5 to 7 minutes for the first side and about 3 to 5 minutes for the second side. Remove from the hot pan and set aside to rest.

Reduce the heat to medium and add the remaining 1 tablespoon (15 g) butter. Once it has melted, drop in the onion, apple, whole bay leaf, thyme and the teaspoon (5 g) of coarse sea salt (use a half teaspoon if choosing a finer-grain salt). Cook and stir for 15 to 20 minutes, or until the volume is reduced by half and the onion and apple turn a light golden brown.

Deglaze the pan with the hard apple cider. This means that when the cider is added to the caramelized onion and apple, the layer of browned bits that have started to form on the bottom of the pan will be lifted up and incorporated into the liquid. Another way to say it is that the glaze of cooked material that has formed on the bottom is removed, or deglazed, when liquid is added to a hot pan with no moisture yet present. Taking this step recycles "browned food bits" stuck to the pan into flavor gems for the sauce.

Return the seared pork loin chops to the pan and nestle them down into the onion mixture. Cover the pan, reduce the temperature to medium low and braise for 30 minutes, or until the internal temperature of the pork reaches 160°F (71°C) for medium-well doneness. Remove and discard the bay leaf.

Allow the pork to rest for 5 to 10 minutes in the pan (but off the heat) before serving or slicing. To serve the pork, transfer each chop to a plate or serving dish, mound a portion of the onion and apples on top of each chop and drizzle with the preferred amount of braising liquid to finish. Chopped fresh Italian flat-leaf parsley makes a lovely garnish, if desired.

BALSAMIC BACON BRUSSELS BITES

I love this recipe because you can make exactly what you need and nothing goes to waste. While I adore these little bites as an appetizer, I found them surprisingly delicious reheated and served with eggs for breakfast. Whether you're looking for an interesting addition to your small-bites party spread, a creative side for grilled steak or a savory brunch item, these Balsamic Bacon Brussels Bites are just the thing!

Serves 6 to 8

---

12 large Brussels sprouts

2 tbsp (30 mL) balsamic vinegar

½ tsp dried thyme

¼ tsp ground black pepper

½ tsp garlic powder

5 or 6 slices of bacon (free of added sugar, preservatives and gluten)

Preheat the oven to 400°F (204°C).

Trim the ends of the Brussels sprouts, just enough to remove the excess core without cutting into the leaves much. Then halve the sprouts lengthwise.

In a shallow dish, combine the balsamic vinegar, thyme, pepper and garlic powder. Add the halved sprouts to the vinegar mixture and gently but thoroughly toss to coat. The more the vinegar mixture can soak into the layers of the sprouts the better, so spoon it directly into the cut sides, too.

When it comes to wrapping the sprouts in bacon, work one slice at a time, one sprout at a time. Lay down a slice of bacon, then grab a Brussels sprout. The bacon constricts when it cooks, so it's important to loosely wrap it over the Brussels sprout to get an accurate measurement and then trim at that point. Continue working through the bacon and sprouts until the sprouts are gone. I'm sure you can come up with a way to use any leftover trimmed bacon....

To secure the bacon, be sure that the cut is squarely under the flat side of the sprout when placed on a baking sheet. There's no need to use a toothpick to secure the bacon; however, if you'd like to serve these bites on a skewer, now is the time to do that. Skewer so that the flat side of the sprout remains against the baking sheet.

Bake for 20 to 23 minutes for crisp bacon and perfectly roasted Brussels sprouts.

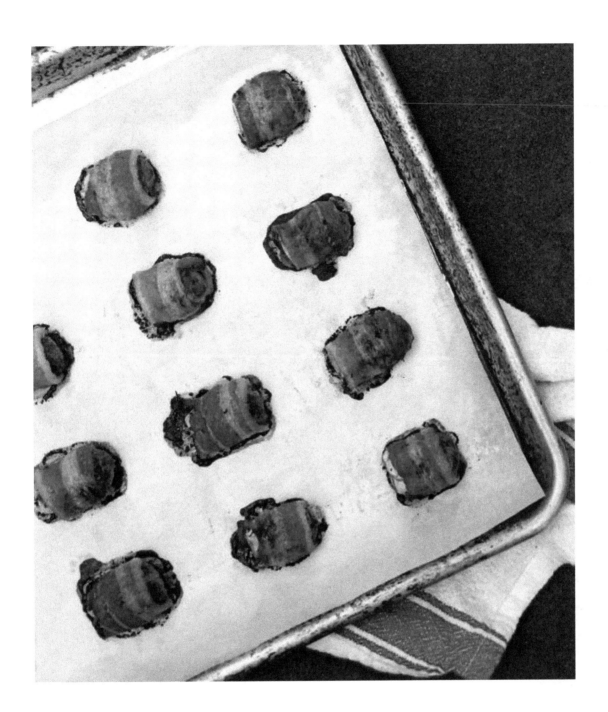

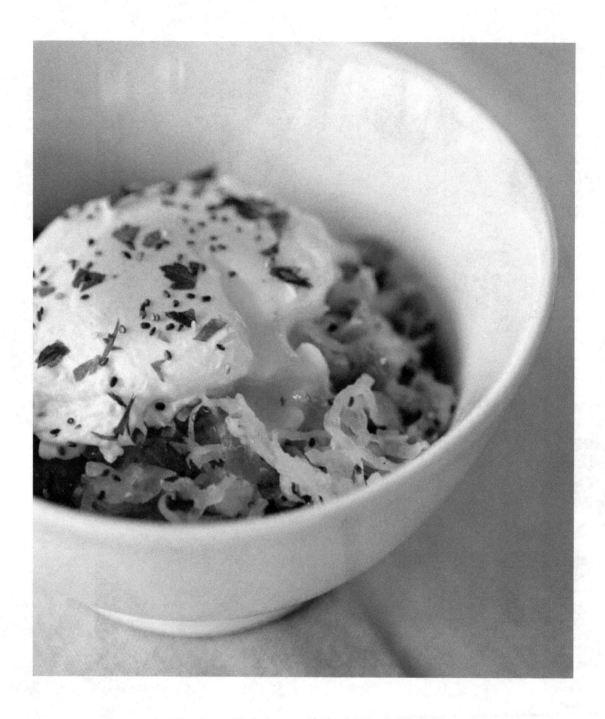

DECONSTRUCTED SPAGHETTI SQUASH CARBONARA

My goal was to make this as easy as possible without sacrificing flavor or adding things that are no-no's (sorry, no Parmesan to be found here). The only real deconstructed element is the poached egg in place of scrambled. I'm a fan of runny eggs, but the whole raw scrambled egg sauce that allegedly cooks from the heat of the pasta has me kind of squeamish. Poaching gives control over the doneness of the egg, so I know the whites are cooked and the yolk is creamy.

Spoiler Alert: To send this over the moon, I fry thinly sliced garlic in reserved bacon fat and then toss in the spaghetti squash. You'll get incredible depth of flavor through this step! Be careful, though, because garlic burns easily. So keep your spaghetti squash close and your tongs closer.

Serves 4

---

1 spaghetti squash (harvested strands equal about 3 cups [1.3 kg])

8 to 10 slices bacon

1 tablespoon (15 mL) white vinegar

4 to 6 eggs (1 or 2 per person)

4 garlic cloves, sliced

1 tsp (5 mL) white wine vinegar

¼ cup (15 g) sliced green onions

1 tbsp (4 g) chopped flat-leaf parsley

Sea salt and pepper, to taste

Chia seeds, for garnish (optional)

Preheat the oven to 375°F (190°C). To make the spaghetti squash, slice it lengthwise down the center, remove the seeds and roast cut side down for 40 minutes. Turn cut side up when roasting is complete and allow to cool slightly before harvesting the strands with a fork by scraping with the grain until the squash is cleaned. Set aside for later. Allow to drain, if possible.

Brown the bacon slices in a skillet, set aside to drain and reserve the fat in a separate container. (You should have about ¼ cup [60 mL] of bacon drippings.) Chop the bacon into bite-size bits (You should have enough to yield 1 cup [225 g] of loosely packed bacon bits.) Set aside.

To make the poached eggs, in a medium saucepan, bring 4 cups (948 mL) of water to a boil with the white vinegar mixed into the water.

Working with one egg at a time, crack it into a small bowl or ramekin. Create a whirlpool in the simmering water and gently slide the egg into the center of it. Allow the egg to poach for 3 minutes, then remove with a slotted spoon. Place on a paper towel to drain the liquid from the egg.

In a clean skillet, heat the reserved bacon drippings over medium-high heat. When it has come to temp, place the garlic into the fat and gently stir. Garlic burns very easily, so be attentive at this step. As soon as the garlic has some color, reduce the heat to medium and add the spaghetti squash, tossing together right away. Moving quickly will save your garlic and give your pasta unique flavor. And heads up: Few things smell better than garlic fried in bacon fat.

Once the spaghetti squash is coated in fat and garlic, add in the white wine vinegar, chopped bacon, green onions and the parsley. Toss to combine and let simmer for just a few minutes more.

To serve, place the desired amount of spaghetti squash on a plate. Top with any extra bacon bits, green onions, parsley and 1 (or 2) of the reserved poached eggs. I like to add a little bit of Celtic sea salt and fresh cracked black pepper at this point as well. If you have chia seeds on hand, sprinkle a bit of those over the dish to garnish.

Break open the yolk to create a silky, rich sauce for your Paleo Carbonara and dig in!

PORK TACOS 101

A handful of ingredients, a blend of basic spices and a little water. That's all it will take to make 101-level pork tacos. This is a bare-bones recipe for your taco springboarding pleasure. Keep it simple with this, or get creative to make it your own. Either way, you can't go wrong.

Serves 6 to 8

---

1 tbsp (15 g) lard (tallow, duck fat, avocado oil and ghee will also work)

3 lb (1.4 kg) boneless pork shoulder or butt

1 batch Taco Seasoning Blend (here)

1 tsp (5 g) coarse sea salt

1 cup (150 g) diced onion

4 cloves garlic, crushed

2 cups (400 g) diced fresh organic tomatoes

½ cup (118 mL) water

Heat a Dutch oven (or other heavy-bottomed stockpot with a lid) over medium-high heat and melt the lard.

Trim the pork into 4- to 5-inch (10- to 13-cm) cubed portions and season liberally with the seasoning blend and sea salt. I like to leave the thick fat attached, but if you prefer to remove it, do so prior to seasoning.

Sear the seasoned pork in the melted lard, working in batches so as not to overcrowd the pan. Attempting to sear too many pieces at once will result in essentially steaming and boiling the meat rather than yielding that golden brown crust we're after. Take your time, it's worth it. Sear every edge of the meat, then set aside.

Replenish the fat in the pan if needed, and add the onion and garlic. Cook and stir until the garlic is fragrant, then add the tomatoes plus the water. Bring to a boil, then immediately reduce the heat to a simmer. Add the seared pork back to the pan and nestle it down into the braising liquid. Cover the Dutch oven and allow to simmer for 2 hours uninterrupted.

When the pork falls away easily with a gentle press from the back of a fork, remove the meat from the Dutch oven and set aside to rest. Increase the temperature to boil the braising liquid, which will concentrate the flavor and reduce the liquid into a thick taco sauce. Boil until that consistency is achieved. This should take less than 10 minutes.

Meanwhile, shred the pork and discard any large pieces of fat that did not render. Once the sauce has reduced, return the shredded pork to the pan and mix together. It's ready to serve!

MUSHROOM SKILLET LASAGNA

This skillet lasagna has more of an earthy flavor to it thanks to the portobellos and chard. It's a refreshing change to the plethora of Paleo bolognese recipes in circulation these days. Serve this dish with roasted spaghetti squash or even just in a bowl with a spoon like a hearty stew. It's satisfying either way.

Serves 4 to 6

---

2 portobello mushrooms

2 to 3 tbsp (30 to 45 mL) extra virgin olive oil

12 oz (340 g) ground Italian pork sausage

1 medium yellow onion, diced

3 cloves garlic, chopped

1 batch Italian Seasoning Blend (here)

1 tsp (5 g) sea salt

3 cups (300 g) chopped red chard (leaves only)

1 (14.5 oz [411 g]) can organic diced tomatoes

1 (15 oz [425 g]) can organic tomato sauce

Start by cleaning the portobellos. Grab the portobello caps and clean off any dirt using a dry kitchen towel. *Resist the temptation to wet the towel.* If you were to use a wet towel, the mushroom would absorb the moisture like a sponge; *resist.* Start from the top center of the cap and gently brush toward the outer edge. That's it.

Use a spoon to remove the gills and stems, then slice the caps into half-inch-wide (1-cm) strips. Cut those strips in half and set aside.

Heat a large, high-sided skillet over medium-high heat and add the olive oil. When the oil comes to temp, meaning that it is glossy and moves easily when tilted from side to side, start adding the meat and veggies. Crumble in the ground Italian sausage and drop in the portobello slices, onion, garlic, seasoning blend and sea salt. Carefully toss to combine, and cook for about 6 minutes. Add in the red chard and cook for another 3 to 4 minutes. The chard will wilt just in time for the other vegetables and ground pork to finish cooking — everything at this point is fully cooked and ready for the crushed tomatoes. Perfectly timed.

Add the diced tomatoes and canned tomato sauce to the pan and bring to a slow bubble. Then reduce the temperature to medium low, cover the pan with a secure lid and simmer for 45 minutes. Simmering at a low temperature for this amount of time will enrich the sauce and bring all of the flavors together into one cohesive dish. Give the dish a few slow stirs during that time, but for the most part leave it undisturbed.

Serve the Mushroom Skillet Lasagna over roasted spaghetti squash (which incidentally will have sufficient time in the oven to fully cook while the Skillet Lasagna simmers) or even just in a bowl eaten with a big spoon, no other sides required.

HARD CIDER BRAISED BRATS

I firmly believe that Paleo food is simple food and do my best to put recipes together that reflect this belief. This recipe couldn't be easier or more delicious. Eat this with a heaping side of sauerkraut and some good-quality mustard.

Serves 2 to 4

---

2 to 3 tbsp (30 to 45 g) lard, bacon drippings or coconut oil

4 or 5 brats from pastured pigs

½ white or yellow onion

1 bay leaf

1 (12 oz [355 mL]) bottle hard apple cider (no added sugar or gluten)

To prep, break out your Dutch oven (or any thick-bottomed pot with a fitted lid) and heat it over medium or medium-high heat—whatever will get you a good sear on your brats. Melt your chosen fat and add the brats to the pan.

Once the brats are placed, don't move them around until it's time to turn them over. The goal is to get a deep brown crust on 2 sides before adding the braising liquid. If you're constantly stirring and moving, they won't sear properly. While the brats do their thing for about 5 to 7 minutes per side, slice about a half cup's (75 g) worth of white or yellow onion.

Once the brats are seared, toss in the sliced onion and bay leaf. Give everything a good stir and pour in the hard apple cider. Bring to a boil first before reducing the heat to low and covering the pot. Let braise for 20 to 25 minutes. Remove and discard the bay leaf.

The hard cider reduces into a sweet and tangy sauce, and the lard gives it a silky texture. It's fantastic!

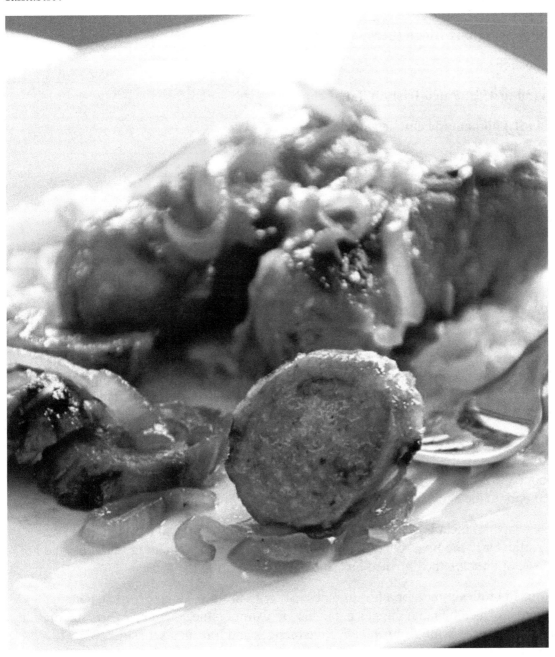

CROCK POT CITRUS CARNITAS

Carnitas are my favorite! A slow cooker makes it ultra convenient to turn out this delicious and affordable dish. A squeeze of fresh citrus juice paired with spicy chipotles in adobo works magic with slow-cooked pork.

Serves 6 to 8

4 to 5 lb (1.8 to 2.3 kg) pork loin roast

1 batch Fajita Seasoning Blend (here)

1 tsp (5 g) kosher salt

2 to 3 tbsp (30 to 45 g) Paleo-friendly fat of choice

2 cups (474 mL) homemade chicken stock

2 tbsp (30 g) tomato paste

1 tbsp (15 g) sauce from chipotles in adobo

3 or 4 crushed garlic cloves

2 navel oranges

1 lime

Slice the roast into 2-inch (25-cm) steaks, going across the grain. Leave all of the fat in place on the roast.

Combine the seasoning blend and kosher salt in a large bowl, one that's large enough to easily toss the pork steaks. Once the seasonings are mixed, add the steaks a couple at a time and coat evenly in the seasonings. At first sight, it doesn't look like it'll be enough seasoning to coat, but it will. Let the meat rest while a skillet comes to temp.

Heat a skillet or large thick-bottomed pan over medium-high heat. Add the fat of your choice. Arrange 2 or 3 steaks in the hot pan at a time, depending on the size, and sear both sides; this will take about 3 to 5 minutes per side. Work in batches to ensure a quick and quality sear. Move the browned pork to the slow cooker to rest. Repeat until all of the pork has been seared.

When the last batch of meat is searing, in a separate bowl, stir together the stock, tomato paste, adobo and garlic. Once the final round of pork is removed, pour the tomato mixture into the hot pan to deglaze, or dissolve the browned bits stuck to the bottom of the pan.

Let this seasoned broth simmer for a few minutes, not only to fully deglaze the pan and incorporate the browned bits into the sauce, but also to warm up the spices and garlic before they joins the pork. While the broth simmers, juice the oranges and lime and set aside.

Pour the broth over the seared pork in the slow cooker. Add the strained citrus juices as well.

Cover and cook on low for 5 hours.

To finish the carnitas, remove the meat from the juices and shred. Discard any larger bits of fat from the pork that did not render in the slow cooker. Transfer the shredded pork to a casserole dish and place under the broiler for a few minutes until the top layer of carnitas has browned and crisped. Remove from the oven and spoon some of the braising liquid over the meat to rehydrate it to your preference, which depends on how you plan to serve the carnitas. For wraps, I leave it on the dry side. However, if I have burrito bowls with cauliflower rice (see here) on the menu, then I will add more juice and let it soak into the cauli-rice for added flavor.

OVEN BARBECUE PORK CHOPS

On my blog, Popular Paleo, I often hesitate to post simple recipes, fearing that they will be disregarded because they are so basic. I have since found that folks actually seek out these straightforward, minimalist recipes. Not every night can be a 5-star meal! With that in mind, Oven Barbecue Pork Chops will likely be a recipe that gets thrown together on those days when you just don't have the energy to prepare yet another Paleo meal and are tempted to order out. Instead, slice an apple and a vegetable or two, grab some berries and pop these chops in the oven. It may not be fancy, but I've called it dinner more than once.

Serves 2 to 4

---

1 batch BBQ Seasoning Blend (here)

½ tsp kosher salt

4 bone-in pork chops

Preheat the oven to 400°F (204°C).

Blend the ingredients called for in the BBQ Seasoning Blend recipe on here, plus the kosher salt.

Lay the pork chops in a nonstick roasting pan, pat both sides dry with a disposable towel and season both sides liberally with the seasoning mixture.

Roast for 20 to 22 minutes, or until the chops reach an internal temperature of 145°F (63°C). Allow the pork to rest for at least 5 minutes before slicing so the juices have an opportunity to redistribute throughout the meat and will not be lost all over your plate.

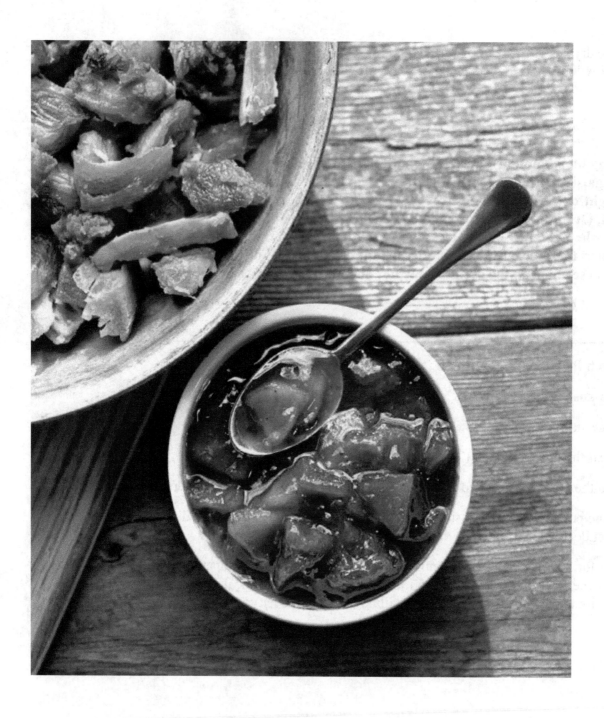

GINGER PEACH PULLED PORK

Unlike carnitas, which are at their best when crisped, Ginger Peach Pulled Pork should be soft, juicy and succulent. To help this pork stay moist during the low-and-slow cooking process and shred easily, I recommend brining it first in a flavorful bath of vinegar, salt, ginger and garlic. This is how you use basic, affordable ingredients to achieve complex, deep flavors in pork that perfectly offset the sweet and spicy tang of fresh ginger peach chutney.

Eat this on top of a baked sweet potato with Bollywood Slaw (here) on the side and watch people disbelieve you've just served a full Paleo meal.

Serves 6 to 8

FOR THE PORK

4 lb (1.8 kg) boneless pork shoulder

1 batch Indian Seasoning Blend (here)

1 tsp (5 g) kosher salt

FOR THE BRINE

½ cup (118 mL) apple cider vinegar

¼ cup (55 g) kosher salt

1 inch (2.5 cm) gingerroot, peeled and sliced into coins

3 cloves garlic, crushed

Water to cover

FOR THE CHUTNEY

1 lb (454 g) ripe peaches (about 4)

½ cup (75 g) diced white or yellow onion

1 inch (2.5 cm) gingerroot, peeled

¼ cup (60 mL) apple cider vinegar

2 tbsp (30 g) coconut palm sugar

¼ tsp kosher salt

⅛ tsp fresh nutmeg

2 grinds of black pepper

Pinch of red-pepper flakes

¼ cup (60 mL) water

This recipe starts with brining the boneless pork shoulder. I like to use a large stockpot with a lid for my brines; however, others have found success with the basin of their slow cookers (not the full unit!) or even a large bucket that you are able to cover. Choose your vessel and prepare the following:

Place the pork shoulder in the pot. Add the apple cider vinegar, kosher salt, gingerroot and garlic. Pour in enough cold water to cover the pork by 2 to 3 inches (5 to 8 cm). Place the lid on the pot and place in the refrigerator for a minimum of 12 hours and up to 24 hours.

To prepare the pork, remove it from the brine and set on a clean work surface such as a butcher's block or cutting board. Use disposable towels to pat the pork dry, and then allow it to rest in the open air while the seasonings are combined. Preheat the oven to 300°F (149°C).

Mix together the spices listed on here for Indian Seasoning Blend plus the kosher salt. Rub this mixture all over the dried pork shoulder and place in a large roasting pan with the fatty layer of the pork facing up. Slow roast the pork, uncovered, for 5 hours.

While the pork is in the oven, prepare the Ginger Peach Chutney. Start by choosing ripe peaches, which should peel easily without needing to be blanched. Select peaches that should be eaten that day; they will be soft (more like a banana than an apple) and fragrant. Peel the peaches, discard the pits and dice. There should be about 3 cups (725 g) of diced peaches, give or take. Place the diced peaches in a medium saucepan.

To the peaches, add the onion, gingerroot, apple cider vinegar, coconut palm sugar, kosher salt, nutmeg, black pepper, red-pepper flakes and water. Stir to combine and place over medium heat until the mixture bubbles, about 5 minutes. Reduce the heat to a simmer and cover. Allow the chutney to simmer for an hour, stirring occasionally.

The chutney is ready when most of the peaches have broken down into a rich, thick sauce. Remove and discard the gingerroot. Allow the chutney to rest at room temperature while the pork shoulder finishes.

After 5 hours, the pork should be ready for shredding. Take it out of the oven and allow it to rest for 10 to 15 minutes at room temperature. Remove any unrendered fat and discard it. Shred the pork (by hand works just fine), returning the meat to the roasting pan as you work. Once the pork is fully shredded, pour the ginger peach chutney over it and combine with the pan juices.

Serve immediately either as a main dish or on top of baked sweet potatoes. This dish makes excellent leftovers!

GRILLED PORK WITH SPICY APRICOT BBQ SAUCE

Rethink BBQ sauce with this combination of exotic, yet accessible, spices and sweet dried apricots. The next time you find pork loin chops on sale, remember this easy recipe that delivers big flavors!

Serves 4

FOR THE SAUCE

1 cup (150 g) diced white or yellow onion

4 cloves garlic, minced

6 whole dried apricots

1 heaping tsp (7 g) finely grated gingerroot

½ tsp ground cinnamon

1 tsp (5 g) ground cumin

½ tsp coarse sea salt

2 tbsp (30 mL) extra virgin olive oil

1 cup (237 mL) water

FOR THE PORK

4 pork loin chops

Salt and black pepper, to taste

Pull the pork loin chops out of the fridge and allow them to rest at room temperature for about 15 minutes, or essentially the time it takes to prepare the sauce.

For the sauce, combine all of the listed ingredients except the water in a medium saucepan and place on a cold burner. Turn the burner to medium and allow it to come to temp. After about 3 minutes, the oil should be hot and the onion should start sizzling. Cook for 5 to 7 minutes, stirring often.

Add the water to the pan to deglaze—a process where the liquid will actually "lift" the brown bits stuck to the bottom of the pan and incorporate them into the sauce as additional flavor. Simmer for 4 to 5 minutes, or until all of the lifted bits from the bottom are absorbed and the liquid is smooth.

Transfer the ingredients to a food processor or a high-speed blender and puree until smooth. Return the puree to the original saucepan and set it aside for later.

For the pork, the first step is to preheat the grill while the pork is prepared.

Trim the excess fat from the pork loin chops. This cut is a pork tenderloin that has been sliced into thick steaks—great for grilling! Bone-in pork chops can be used as well. Generously season both sides of the pork with salt and black pepper.

When the grill has come to temp (about 450°F or 232°C), place the loin chops down on the grate over indirect heat, cover with the lid and walk away. Resist the temptation to poke, prod or peek at the grilling meat too much. Allow the magic of the grill to work on these delicious cuts of lean pork.

After 5 to 6 minutes, turn the pork to the other side. If the pork doesn't easily lift away from the grate, let it go for another minute or so. Meat tells us when it is ready to be turned because it will easily release from the hot grill when the time is right.

Once you've turned the chops, grab the waiting sauce and baste the cooked side of the pork with it. Slather it on as generously as you prefer.

Continue grilling the second side for about 6 minutes, or until the internal temperature of the pork reaches 145°F (63°C). Then turn the grill temperature to as low as possible (or ensure the pork is situated at the coolest location of the grill) and turn the pork back over and baste the unsauced side. Close the lid again and let rest for 1 minute. Then turn the pork again, apply yet another layer of sauce and transfer to a serving dish.

Transfer any unused sauce to a serving dish so your guests can add extra during dinner.

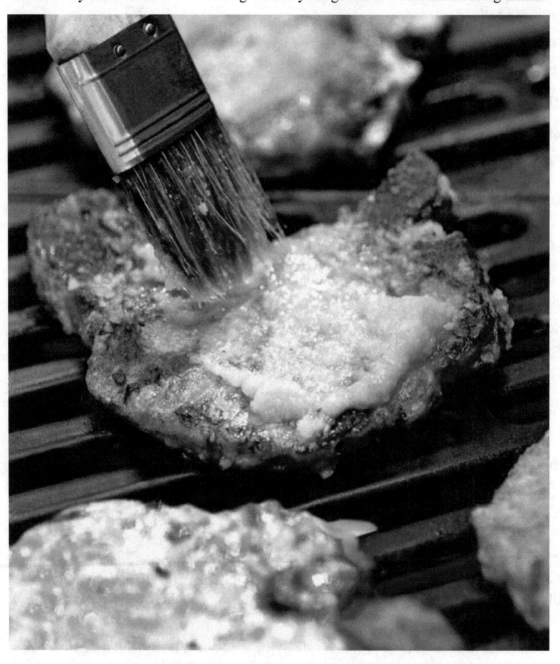

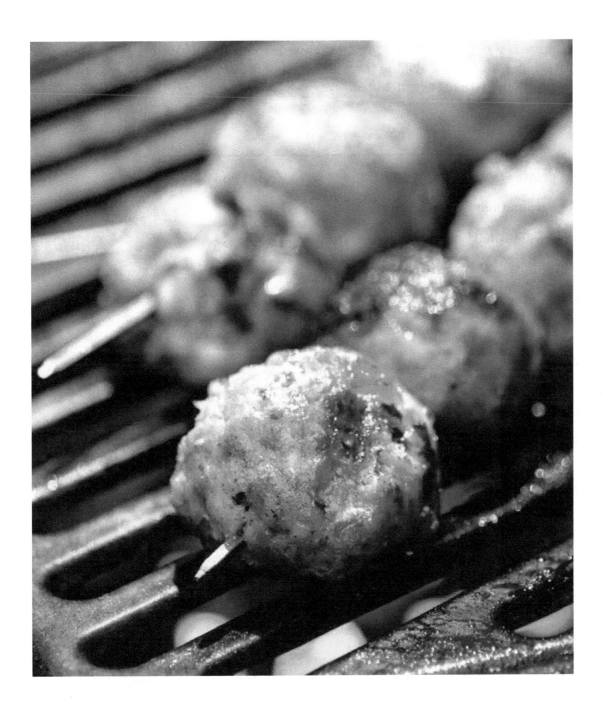

POT STICKER MEATBALLS

I'm part Chinese, and while I don't always care for traditional Chinese fare (a girl can handle only so many fish cheeks and soups filled with obscure fungi), I do enjoy a good dumpling. So when thinking about how to make those dumplings Paleo and affordable, both on the wallet and on time, it seemed like a no-brainer to just cook everything but the noodle and call it a meatball. Turns out, it was a good idea indeed.

There are 2 options when it comes to cooking these meatballs. While baking is always a convenient option, I found that grilling them kabob style was really worth the extra effort. Instructions for both methods are included.

Serves 4 to 6

---

8 oz (227 g) prawns (31 to 40 per pound [454 g] size), peeled and deveined

12 oz (340 g) ground pork

½ cup (115 g) finely diced canned water chestnuts

¼ cup (15 g) thinly sliced green onions

2 cloves garlic, minced

½ inch (1 cm) gingerroot, peeled and finely diced

3 tbsp (45 mL) coconut aminos

If you are baking the meatballs, preheat the oven to 400°F (204°C). If you'd like to grill the meatballs (which I recommend), then preheat the grill to 500°F (260°C).

Prepare all of the ingredients as directed. Then grab the peeled/deveined prawns and roughly chop into small pieces. If you've never made Chinese dumpling filling before, this will admittedly look a little strange. Go with it, though. I promise there is a good reason for chopping up perfectly good prawns.

Place all of the ingredients in a mixing bowl and combine them by hand. Unfortunately, there really isn't a better tool than your hands when it comes to mixing ingredients into ground meat.

Once this is combined, use a quarter-cup (60-mL) measuring cup to scoop out equal portions of the meatball mixture. Working one portion at a time, roll between your palms to form an even meatball and place it on a baking sheet lined with parchment or a silicone mat. You'll notice that the mixture is quite loose; this is intentional. Keep moving forward.

If you'd like to bake the meatballs, pop them in the oven and bake for 23 to 26 minutes. If you'd like to grill the meatballs, I recommend skewering them first. Arrange 3 or 4 meatballs in a row on the baking sheet and skewer by poking the skewer straight through the center of the row. Repeat until they're all loaded up. Carry the baking sheet over to the grill and use a metal spatula to help transfer the skewers to the grill. The pork mixture is somewhat fragile raw, so do not attempt to move the skewers around without supporting the meatballs.

Grill for about 15 to 18 minutes, or until the pork is no longer pink. Be sure to rotate the skewers 2 or 3 times while grilling so they cook evenly on all sides.

These meatballs are fantastic on their own or with a host of Asian-inspired sauces. From faux-peanut sauces to spicy soy alternatives and even some sweet chili sauces, pick a favorite and enjoy these Pot Sticker Meatballs as an appetizer, snack or casual meal.

TANGY APRICOT PULLED PORK

Tangy, sweet, salty pork … I want to write it a love song. A couple of basic pantry ingredients plus a handful of dried apricots that are easy to pick up in the raw bulk section of your local health food store transform this basic piggy into a show-stopping swine! This is how you impress your dinner guests without breaking the bank.

Serves 8

---

6 dried apricots (no added sugars or preservatives)

1 tsp (5 g) coarse sea salt

2 tbsp (30 mL) white wine vinegar

1 clove garlic

5 to 6 grinds black pepper

2 tbsp (30 mL) Dijon mustard

1 tbsp (15 mL) water

5 lb (2.3 kg) boneless pork shoulder

Preheat the oven to 300°F (149°C).

Soak the apricots in hot water for 15 minutes, or until softened. Drain the water and toss the apricots into a food processor. Add the salt, vinegar, garlic, black pepper, Dijon mustard and water and pulse to break down the apricots a bit before letting the mixture puree. Intermittently stop and use a rubber spatula to scrape down the sides. A high-powered blender also works great for whipping up the glaze.

Completely coat the pork shoulder in the apricot glaze and set in a high-sided roasting pan with the fat layer facing up. Cover with foil and slow roast for 5 hours. The pork should be no cooler than 165°F (74°C) internally, but will likely be over 200°F (93°C) after 5 hours. That is perfect.

At this point, you have two options. Either remove the pork from the pan and shred as is with a soft, saucy glaze (discarding the large pieces of unrendered fat), or baste the shoulder with pan juices, then transfer to another (dry) roasting pan and return the pork to the oven for an additional 15 to 20 minutes at 375°F (190°C) to crisp the outside. No matter which option you choose, allow the pork to rest for 10 minutes or so before shredding.

SLOW COOKER VARIATION: If you're not able to babysit your oven all day, this recipe works great in a slow cooker! Prepare the glazed pork as directed, but place in a large slow cooker instead of the preheated oven. Set the temperature to low and cook for 7 to 8 hours. Shred and serve in the same manner.

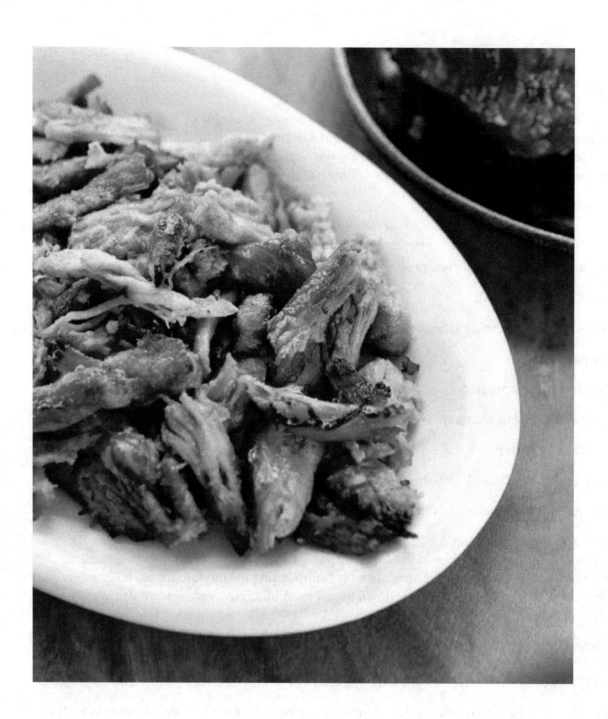

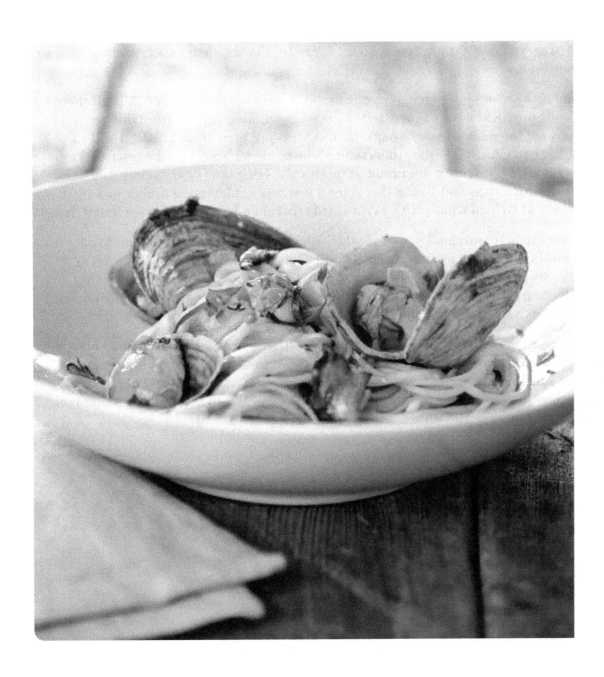

Consider the practice of foraging in the Paleolithic Era for a moment. Foods were seasonal and regional. It's a totally modern concept that we could have whatever ingredient we want and at any time of year—not that I'm complaining or anything. And now that we have access, we want affordable access. But here's the way I see it: sourcing quality, affordable foods still, even all these years later, comes down to geography.

I currently live in a region with rich soil, thanks to some volcanoes nearby. We have thriving farmers' markets here as a result! There was a time when I lived sandwiched in between enormous mountain ranges and enjoyed wild game for the price of a hunting license. And now, as I look out onto the beautiful Puget Sound of Washington state, fresh, reasonably priced seafood is at my fingertips. Ultimately, it's a trade-off. Look around you. What's local? Make that your primary protein source. And if, after surveying the immediate area, you don't come across a vast ocean by chance, then let's talk about how to get you some seafood.

Since taking on a second job to pay for your family's weekly allotment of fish is off the table, my most practical advice is to offset the costs by making super-affordable recipes on the other days of the week. Hearty Spaghetti and Meatball Stew (here), Paleo Hotdish (here) and Braised Chicken Fajitas (here) can all be made for less than the price of fresh fish for four and can provide a minimum of two meals. Then take your savings and enjoy some Zoodles with Clams and Bacon (here) for a luscious Friday night dinner or a light weekend lunch of Grilled Clams with Fried Garlic (here) and Summer Prawn Salad (here).

When it comes time to purchase your fish, shellfish and the like, check out your local wholesale retailer. Bulk is king no matter if you're talking about a sack of potatoes or a pack of flash-frozen fresh halibut fillets. Also, there are several websites that will ship fresh, locally sourced seafood overnight to your doorstep no matter where you call home. Hop online, search for a company that you like and place a bulk order with them.

Lastly, while we know that fresh is ideal, remember there are also quality canned options available for wild, sustainably sourced seafood. Canned tuna and sardines are great for lunches and snacks! So while we tend to think about a nice fresh fillet for dinner, it's equally as good to pile up canned sardines, hard-cooked eggs, olives and fresh tomato on a bed of greens for an easy and affordable seafood salad at lunchtime.

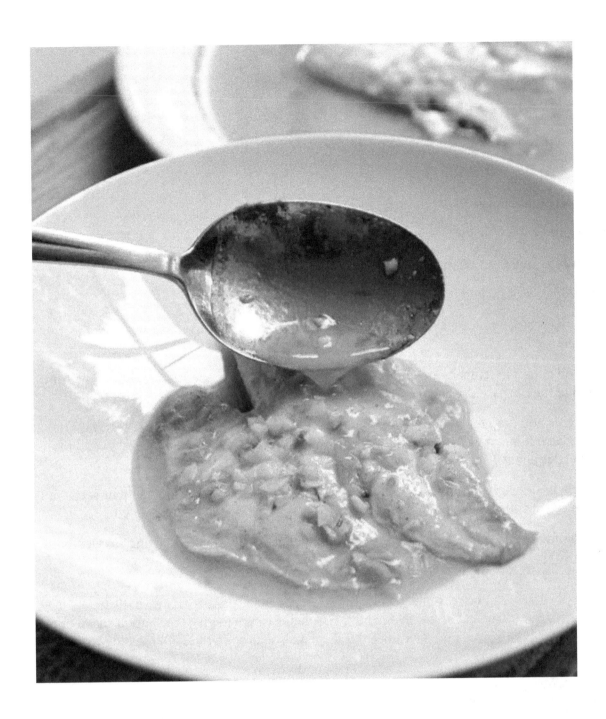

CUBAN TILAPIA IN MOJO SAUCE

Mojo sauce is just about one of the easiest sauces you will ever make. It is light yet distinct, making it a perfect partner for white flaky fish. Since it can also be made in advance and stored in the refrigerator for a few days, this recipe is ideal to incorporate into bulk food prep day. Make the sauce on Saturday or Sunday, store in the fridge, then pour it over fresh tilapia on Tuesday or Wednesday for a fast and easy dinner.

Serves 2

FOR THE SAUCE

½ cup (118 mL) extra virgin olive oil

6 cloves garlic

1 red grapefruit

1 lime

1 tsp (5 g) ground cumin

½ tsp sea salt

1 to 1.5 lb (454 to 683 g) fresh, skinless tilapia fillets

Preheat the oven to 425°F (218°C).

Start by preparing the mojo sauce. Pour the olive oil into a small saucepan and warm over medium heat.

While the oil comes to temperature, mince the garlic and juice the grapefruit and lime. The fruit juices should together yield 1 cup (237 mL) of liquid.

Once the oil is hot, drop the minced garlic into the saucepan and stir immediately. Garlic burns quickly, so keep it moving (though gently, so the oil isn't splashed) and be prepared to add the fresh juice after about 30 to 45 seconds.

Carefully pour in the grapefruit and lime juice through a strainer or sieve so no pulp or seeds fall into the sauce, and stir. The bubbling will calm once the juices are fully incorporated.

Add the cumin and sea salt. Stir again and cook for another 2 to 3 minutes, stirring frequently.

Remove the sauce from the burner and allow to cool while the fish is prepared.

*Note that this sauce can be made in advance and stored in an airtight container in the refrigerator for a few days at this point once fully cooled. Be sure to give the sauce a shake or a good mix before pouring over the fish since the sauce will separate a little after resting that long.

For the fish, rinse the tilapia under cold water and pat dry with a disposable towel.

Lay the fish in a nonstick baking dish in a single layer and cover with the mojo sauce. Only 1 cup (237 mL) of sauce is necessary for 1 pound (454 g) of fish, whereas the full batch of sauce should be used if you end up with 1 ½ pounds (683 g) of tilapia.

Bake the fish, uncovered, for 30 minutes, or until it flakes easily. Serve hot.

GRILLED CLAMS WITH FRIED GARLIC

Thinly sliced fried garlic is my family's secret weapon for basic seafood dishes when we don't want to put much effort into dinner. We typically pour hot oil with fried garlic and fresh chilies over whole baked fish to crisp the skin and sear the inner meat. However, I've

found that the same approach works unbelievably well with fresh grilled steamer clams. Serve this dish as an appetizer for two or a main course for one.

Serves 2

---

1 lb (454 g) steamer clams

¼ cup (60 g) grass-fed butter or ghee

2 or 3 cloves garlic, thinly sliced

⅛ tsp crushed red-pepper flakes

1 tbsp (10 g) chopped fresh flat-leaf parsley

Pinch of coarse-grain sea salt, such as Celtic

Place the clams in a colander and scrub under running water to remove grit and sand as best as possible.

Grill the clams over direct heat in a single layer. Depending on the size of the clam, it could take as little as 3 minutes or as much as 10 to open; opening is the cue that it's fully cooked and ready to remove from the heat. If a clam hasn't opened within 5 minutes, shift it to a hot spot on the grill and give it a few more minutes. If it still doesn't open, it needs to be tossed; it's bad.

Once the clams have all opened, place in a serving dish and cover while the sauce is prepared.

For the sauce, place the butter or ghee in a small saucepan and heat over medium-high heat. When it has melted, and even sizzles a little bit, add the garlic slices and red-pepper flakes. Right away, start stirring and moving the garlic. Garlic goes from sweet and golden to bitter and burnt in seconds, so keep a watchful eye over it and do not stop moving the slices. Finding the sweet spot will take between 2 and 3 minutes, so as soon as the garlic turns a deep yellow, pull the pan off the heat and spoon the sauce over the clams. The residual heat will finish the garlic to a crisp, perfect golden brown.

Finish the clams by sprinkling with the parsley and a pinch of coarse-grain sea salt. Enjoy right away!

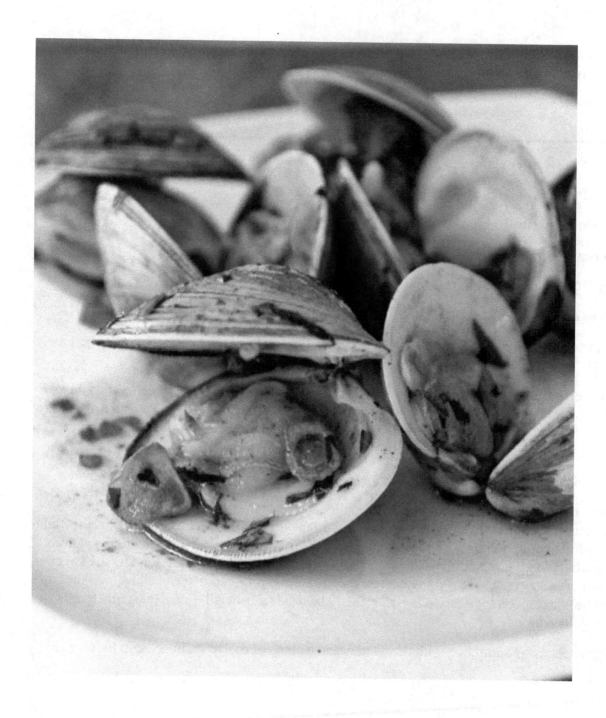

ASIAN-STYLE PRAWNS

I grew up in a Chinese-Italian household; this recipe is what we considered fast food. Since our home was rarely without a supply of fresh garlic, green onions and cilantro, quickly cooking some prawns was a default dinner for us. Thanks to coconut aminos, this recipe easily converts to Paleo, making it one of our regular dinners in my home now as well.

I recommend purchasing prawns that have already been peeled and deveined. It's a huge time saver that doesn't add much additional cost. Acknowledging that your time is just as valuable as your money, save yourself a step and choose prawns that do not require additional preparation prior to assembling the actual recipe.

Serves 2 to 3

---

1 lb (454 g) wild-caught prawns (31 to 40 per pound [454 g] size), peeled and deveined

2 cloves garlic

2 to 3 green onions

Small bunch cilantro

¼ cup (60 mL) coconut aminos

2 tsp (10 mL) coconut oil

Sesame seeds, for garnish

Thaw the prawns if still frozen by running them under cool water until they become soft. Even lukewarm water could potentially start to cook the prawns if left under the water long enough, so keep it cold when it comes to defrosting prawns.

Lay the thawed prawns in a single layer on a disposable towel to drain as much moisture away from them as possible. While those dry out, prepare the other ingredients.

Finely mince the garlic, thinly slice a quarter cup (15 g) of green onions and roughly chop about one-third of a cup (26 g) of cilantro. Measure out the coconut aminos as well.

Put the prawns in a mixing bowl and combine with the coconut aminos and minced garlic. Allow to rest again at room temperature so the prawns absorb the flavors.

Heat a large skillet over medium-high heat and melt the coconut oil. When the oil has come to temp (it is glossy and moves easily when tilted from side to side), arrange a single layer of prawns in the pan. Prawns don't require much time on the heat to cook through, about 2 to 3 minutes on one side and a minute or so on the other. When the prawns just turn pink, transfer them to a temporary holding dish. Carryover cooking will finish the job, giving you tender prawns. Continue working in batches until all of the prawns are cooked.

Turn off the heat and return the prawns (and any juices that have drained while resting) to the pan. Add in the green onions and cilantro and toss to combine.

Transfer to a serving dish and sprinkle with some toasted sesame seeds to garnish.

CREOLE BAKED COD

Dinner doesn't get much simpler than this. Pick up some fresh cod, toss it in Creole Seasoning Blend (here) and bake. Throw together an easy vegetable side like Ginger

Carrots (here) or Hard Cider Sprouts (here), or have a batch of Overnight Salad (here) waiting for you, and dinner is done in 30 minutes—and with minimal dishes to clean up!

If you're looking for the kick that comes more from Cajun-style cooking, swap out the Creole Seasoning Blend for Blackening Seasoning Blend (here) and prepare in the same manner. You'll have spicy baked cod waiting for you in minutes.

Serves 2

---

1 batch Creole Seasoning Blend (here)

¼ tsp kosher salt

1 lb (454 g) skinless cod fillets

A few lemon wedges

Preheat the oven to 425°F (218°C). While the oven heats up, mix the seasoning blend together, plus the kosher salt.

Place the cod in a large resealable plastic bag, dump in the seasoning and seal securely. Toss the fish around in the bag to completely coat in the seasoning blend.

Transfer the cod to a nonstick baking dish and bake, uncovered, for 30 minutes, or until the fish flakes easily. Serve with lemon wedges and Homemade Mayo (here) or your favorite Paleo tartar sauce or remoulade.

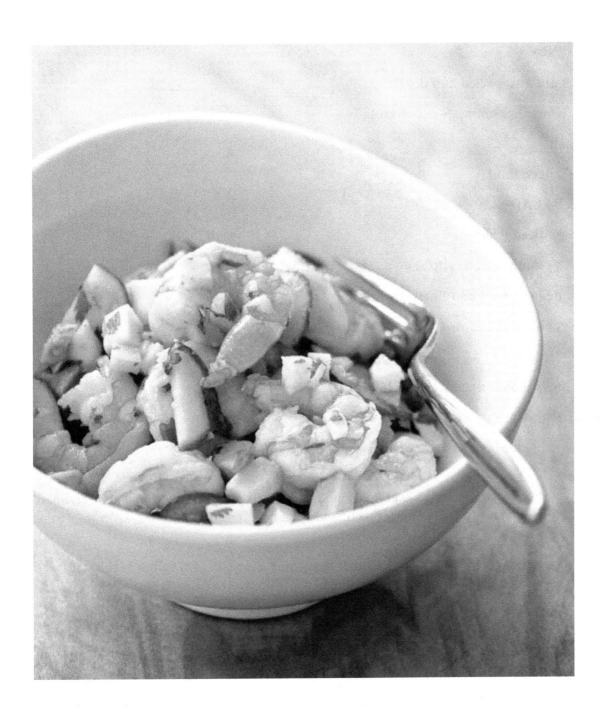

SUMMER PRAWN SALAD

Light, fresh and mayo-free! Exactly what we want in a salad on a hot summer's day. Seasoned prawns are delicious in this recipe, but feel free to substitute leftover shredded chicken or pulled pork or even omit a protein altogether. This salad is flexible without sacrificing flavor.

Serves 4

FOR THE PRAWNS

1 lb (454 g) prawns, peeled and deveined

1 tsp (5 g) House Seasoning Blend (here)

½ tsp sea salt

2 tsp (10 g) coconut oil

FOR THE SALAD

1 cup (225 g) diced jicama

½ cup (115 g) thinly sliced radishes

1 large jalapeño, seeded and finely diced

½ cup (15 g) chopped cilantro

1 avocado, diced

Juice of 2 limes (about a quarter cup [60 mL])

A pinch of coarse-grain sea salt

Start by preparing the prawns so they have a chance to cool while the rest of the salad is compiled.

Set the prawns out on a disposable towel in a single layer so they dry a bit before being seasoned, about 5 minutes. Remove the tails or any bits of shell that may have been missed when they were peeled.

In a bowl, toss the air-dried prawns in the House Seasoning Blend and sea salt to evenly distribute the seasonings.

Heat a sauté pan over medium heat and melt the coconut oil. Once it is hot (the oil is glossy and moves easily across the pan when tilted from side to side), drop in the prawns. Cook and stir for 3 to 5 minutes, or until the prawns are pink and firm. Remove from the heat and set aside to cool while the salad is prepared.

Combine all of the salad ingredients in a large bowl. When the prawns have cooled completely, add them to the salad. Stir once more and serve. This can be stored in the refrigerator for up to 4 hours prior to serving, though refrigeration is not necessary prior to serving.

ZOODLES WITH CLAMS AND BACON

Goodbye, gluten-loaded clams and linguine. Hello, Zoodles with Clams and Bacon! Next time you get a craving for the classic white sauce clam dish, give this one a try instead.

Serves 4

2 lb (908 g) steamer clams

1 cup (237 mL) organic chicken stock

2 tbsp (30 g) grass-fed butter or ghee

3 cloves garlic, minced

1 cup (175 g) chopped cooked bacon

4 (6 inch [15 cm]) zucchini, cut with a spiral slicer into "noodles"

Chopped fresh flat-leaf parsley, for garnish (optional)

Place the steamer clams in a colander and scrub well under running water to remove sand and grit caught in the shells.

Pour the chicken stock into a large, high-sided skillet, add the cleaned steamer clams, cover the pan with a secure lid and turn the temperature to medium-high. After about 5 to 7 minutes the clams should have opened up, indicating they are now cooked; discard any that are not. Clams that don't open after being cooked are bad; toss them.

Remove the clams from the pan, including any that may have fallen out of their shells while cooking, and set aside. Then drain the stock and clam juice into a heatproof jar or bowl and set it aside for later. Do not disturb this. Even though the clams were washed, there may still have been a bit of sand and grit tucked into the shells that was freed when they were cooked. Allowing the juices to rest will let the sand and grit fall to the bottom of the jar or bowl, making it easy to avoid adding them back to the pan in just a few minutes.

While the pan juice rests, harvest the clams from their shells with the exception of 3 or 4 clams, which will be used as a garnish for the finished dish.

Place the same high-sided skillet back on the burner, turn the heat to medium and melt the butter or ghee. Add the garlic, bacon and harvested clams. Cook and stir for 2 to 3 minutes to warm the bacon and cook the garlic.

Next, add the spiral-cut zucchini "noodles" to the pan and toss to combine with the bacon, clams and garlic. Zoodles are easily overcooked when kept on the heat for longer than just a few minutes, so work quickly after they are first tossed in the clam and bacon mixture.

As soon as the mixture is evenly combined, slowly pour in the reserved chicken stock with clam juice—all but the last quarter cup (60 mL). Remember that the sand and grit from the clams has settled to the bottom, so avoid pouring that back into the dish. Discard the remaining amount of liquid.

Toss the zoodles again to evenly coat in the sauce, transfer to a serving dish, top with the reserved 3 or 4 clams from earlier and serve immediately. If you have some fresh flat-leaf parsley on hand, chop a tablespoon or two and sprinkle over the zoodles to garnish.

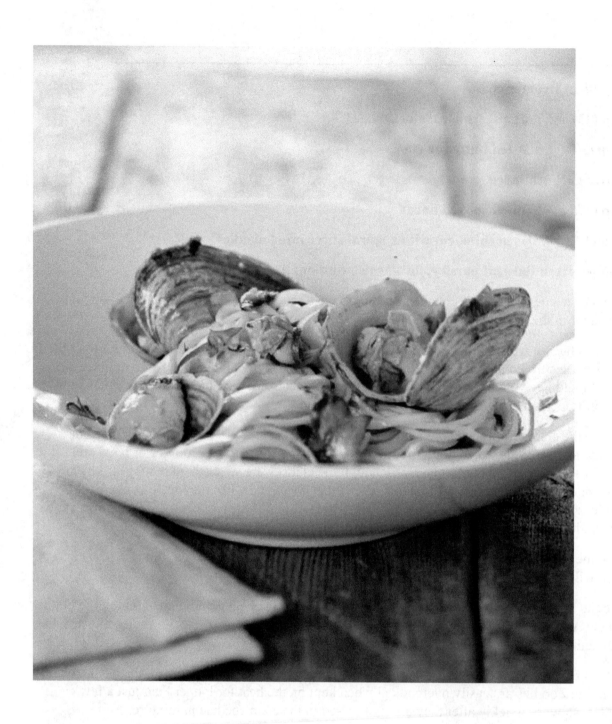

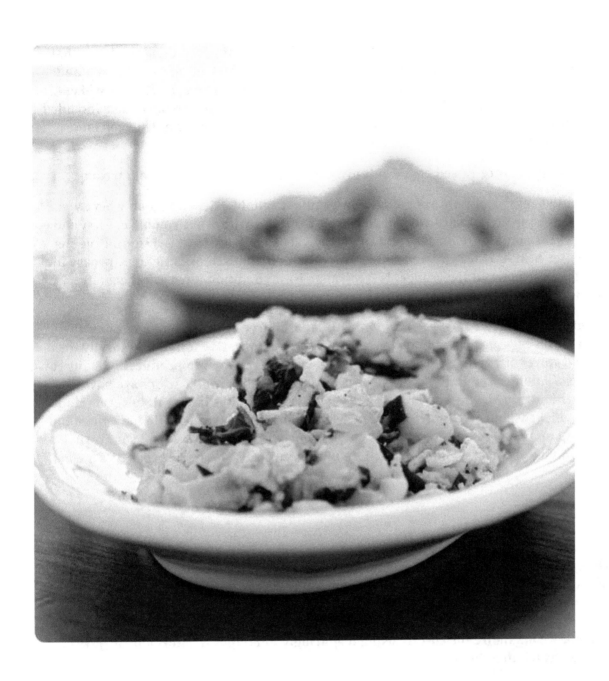

It's no wonder eggs are so popular in Paleo. They are just about the most affordable source of protein available and can be quickly prepared without a high degree of skill. Eggs are also super flexible and go well with a variety of different spices, fats, vegetables and other proteins. From poached with slices of smoked salmon to nestled in a spicy tomato sauce and baked, eggs are an essential food that transcends ethnicities, budgets and cooking abilities.

So what's the catch? Well, you need to know when you're getting ripped off. In a time when people are becoming more health-conscious and concerned about the quality of their food (and their food's food), marketing strategies will abound to capitalize on the underinformed. *Don't be that guy.*

For example, when packaging boasts the all-vegetarian diet they feed their chickens, that's your cue to know those poor birds don't get around much. Chickens are omnivores, and when allowed to mill about in open air and free space (e.g., pasture-raised), they will eat what their genetics dictate. This will include bugs! In order for eggs to have their intended intrinsic nutritional benefits, they must come from chickens that were able to consume their natural diet.

But let's face it, pasture-raised eggs don't grow on trees. Wait. That came out wrong …

Pasture-raised eggs aren't always going to be readily available, depending on where you live and what your lifestyle affords. So do the best you can with what you have. First and foremost, choose organic. Eliminating toxic chemicals from your food is a significant step toward better health. Once you've located grocery stores that sell organic eggs, peruse the cartons for those marked free-range. If free-range isn't an option, then select cage-free. Do your best to avoid general, industrialized eggs.

Think outside the carton and seek out nontraditional sources. While it may be convenient to grab a dozen eggs at the neighborhood chain grocery store, I've found that locally owned health food stores or even smaller markets tend to partner with area producers, selling top-quality eggs. Another fun thing to consider is asking around for folks who have backyard chickens with overachieving egg layers! For example, my yard is too small to accommodate backyard chickens, but I've gotten in contact with folks in my area who do have them but cannot keep up with eating the eggs their chickens produce. I BYOC (bring your own carton) and pass them a few bucks; they give me pasture-raised, organic eggs. It's a win-win.

MAPLE WALNUT SCOTCH EGGS

Scotch eggs are fantastic! Imagine hard-cooked eggs wrapped in delicious sausage and baked until golden brown. This recipe is a spin on the classic way to make them. Chopped walnuts offer added texture to the savory ground pork, and a touch of maple syrup sweetens the deal. While purchasing pure, organic grade B maple syrup can feel like an investment, we maximize the cost by using it sparingly in recipes like this one. Enjoy the flavor and stretch that dollar!

Serves 4 to 6

---

24 oz (680 g) pastured ground pork

2 tbsp (30 mL) pure maple syrup

¼ cup (29 g) chopped walnuts, plus a couple tablespoons (15 g) extra, for garnish

6 hard-cooked eggs

Preheat the oven to 375°F (190°C).

Using your hands, combine the pork, maple syrup and chopped walnuts. Once mixed, divide into 6 even portions.

Grab your plastic wrap. Plastic wrap is the key to making symmetrical, well-rounded Scotch eggs. The sausage easily molds around the egg the way you need it without sticking to your hands in the process.

Lay a sheet of plastic wrap down on a clean, dry work surface. Spread a portion of sausage mixture into a flattened patty in the center of the plastic wrap. Place a hard-cooked egg down on top of that. Lifting up from under the plastic wrap, gently mold the sausage around the egg and seal completely. Once all of the Scotch Eggs have been formed, discard the plastic wrap. Place the Scotch eggs on a nonstick roasting pan or on a baking sheet lined with parchment or a silicone mat.

Top with the extra chopped walnuts. Bake for 40 to 45 minutes. The outside should be a deep brown with the sausage nicely cooked through without being overdone.

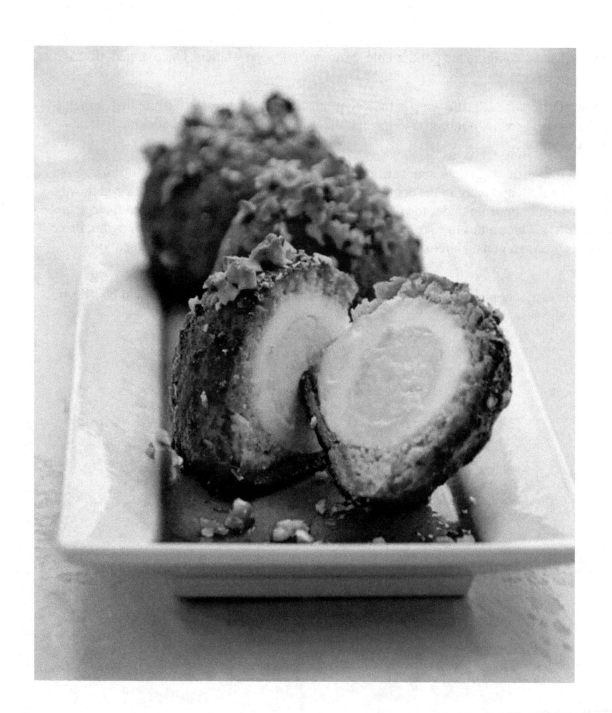

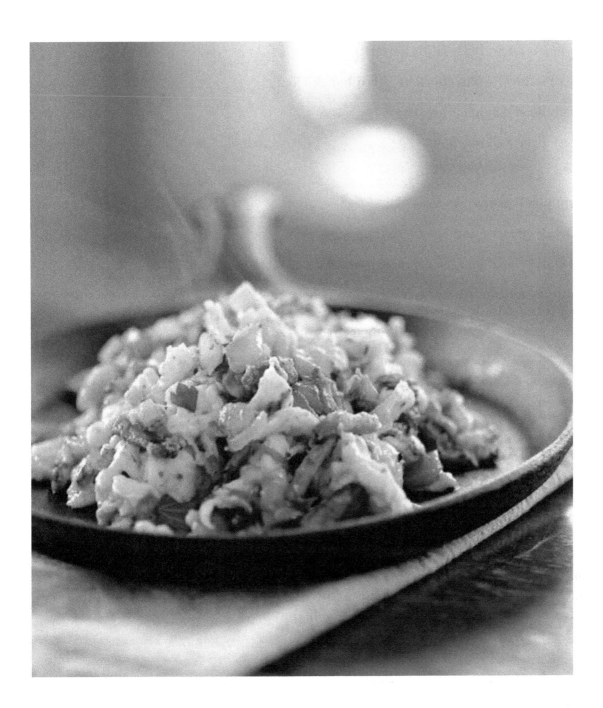

SANTA FE SKILLET

Eggs are a staple in the Paleo diet. I never get tired of finding new ways to eat them for breakfast, lunch or dinner. This skillet of leftover shredded chicken or pulled pork is perfect any time of day and costs only a few bucks to put together. I definitely recommend saving a portion of Tequila Carnitas (here) or Spatchcock Cilantro-Lime Chicken (here) so you can have this delicious skillet for breakfast the next day.

Serves 2 to 3

1 tsp (5 g) Paleo-friendly fat (I prefer lard)

1 cup (250 g) leftover pulled pork or shredded chicken

½ cup (85 g) diced Anaheim peppers

¼ cup (40 g) diced yellow onion

6 eggs

Sea salt and black pepper, to taste

Chopped fresh cilantro and hot sauce (optional)

Heat a skillet over medium heat and melt your preferred fat in the pan.

Cook and stir the leftover pork or chicken, peppers and onion for 5 to 7 minutes, or until the onion is nearly translucent, the peppers are softened and the meat is heated through, or even a little crispy around the edges. Remove from the pan and set aside.

In a medium bowl, whisk the eggs. Replenish some fat in the pan if it looks dry, then pour in the whisked eggs and season with sea salt and pepper. Gently fold and shift the eggs as they begin to set up. When they have some form but are still too wet to consider done, return the meat and veggies to the pan and lightly combine.

After just 2 to 3 additional minutes, the eggs will lose their glossy sheen. They're done cooking! Transfer to a serving dish and enjoy with fresh cilantro and hot sauce, if you choose.

CHILAQUILES

One of my favorite breakfasts is a Tex-Mex dish called Chilaquiles—veggie scramble with cheese and crushed tortilla chips. That version isn't exactly Paleo-friendly, so it's high time we fix that. Make a batch of plantain chips and crush those over the finished product for that classic salty crunch that makes this dish so distinct!

Serves 2 to 3

---

2 cups (450 g) spinach

1 (6 inch [15 cm]) zucchini

2 large white mushroom caps (about 1 cup [75 g])

1 small white or yellow onion

6 organic local eggs

2 tsp (10 g) lard, ghee or coconut oil Salt and black pepper, to taste

A handful of crushed Plantain Chips (here)

Spinach Guacamole Salsa (here) and hot sauce, for serving (optional)

Heat a skillet or heavy-bottomed pan over medium-high heat. Meanwhile, chop the spinach, zucchini and mushrooms, dice the onion and whisk the eggs.

Once the pan is hot, drop in the fat of your choice. When it's glossy and moves easily across the pan when tilted from side to side, add the zucchini, onion and mushrooms. Cook and stir for about 5 to 7 minutes, or until the onion is translucent and the zucchini and mushrooms take on some color. Add the spinach and cook until wilted. Remove the veggies from the pan, replenish some fat if needed and pour in the whisked eggs.

When the eggs have set up a bit (but are far too wet to call done), add the veggies back to the pan and season with salt and pepper. Combine the vegetables with the eggs and continue to cook and stir until the eggs are done. The eggs are ready when the sheen has turned dull and the eggs are fluffy and firm.

When serving, crunch a handful of plantain chips over the top. I love to eat this with Spinach Guacamole Salsa (here) and some hot sauce as well, but that part is up to you.

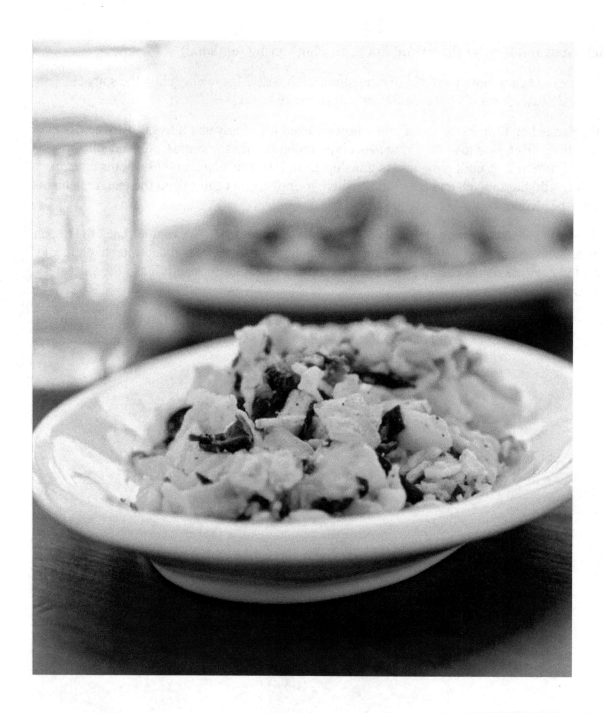

CRAB CAKE FRITTATA

Crab only sounds like a decadent, luxurious ingredient. Canned crab is remarkably affordable—and equally delicious. This frittata maximizes the purchase with a few green onions and eggs for a convenient, economical protein dish that can be eaten any time of day.

Serves 4 to 6

6 to 8 eggs

2 tsp (10 mL) Paleo-friendly fat, such as lard, ghee or extra virgin olive oil

1 cup (230 g) crab meat (if canned, use 2 6 oz [170 g]) cans, drained)

¼ cup (15 g) thinly sliced green onions

Pinch of salt

Black pepper, to taste

Paprika, for garnish (optional)

To start, heat a medium (10 inch [25 cm]) cast-iron skillet (or an oven-safe pan) over medium-high heat.

Beat 6 to 8 eggs, depending on size. Use 6 eggs if they are on the large side; use 8 if somewhat smaller. (Most fresh eggs from backyard chickens, for example, vary more than the eggs found in regular grocery stores.)

Melt your choice of fat in the skillet. Add the drained crab meat and green onions to the hot pan. Season with a pinch of salt and a few grinds of pepper, and cook and stir for 2 to 3 minutes.

Pour the whisked eggs over the crab and green onions. Break up any large clumps of crab so it is evenly distributed among the eggs. This will help the frittata stay intact when sliced. Cook for about 4 minutes undisturbed (without mixing), or until the edges begin to pull away from the sides of the pan without breaking.

Sprinkle a pinch of paprika over the top of the frittata if you'd like it for garnish and transfer to the oven. Place on the rack 3 rungs down from the top, or about 9 inches (23 cm) from the broiler. Turn the broiler on the low setting to cook the top and finish setting the eggs. This should take approximately 5 to 6 minutes. The top of the frittata should be a deep orange to slightly golden, but not browned completely. The frittata should be somewhat firm to the touch and free of any pools of liquid from the beaten eggs.

Turn the oven off, return the pan to the stovetop, cover (foil is fine) and let rest for a minute or two. Resting allows the frittata to loosen from the pan, making service a breeze. Lift the frittata out of the pan and transfer to a cutting board. Slice into 6 wedges and serve with your favorite Paleo cocktail or tartar sauce.

EGGPLANT TOMATO SKILLET

An instant summertime brunch favorite—that is, if you're a fan of creamy, runny yolks. I adore the sauce that is formed right on my plate between the bright tomatoes and savory yolk. It's delicious with every bite of spicy eggplant! I originally came up with this dish to use the leftover half of an eggplant from another recipe I made that didn't require the whole thing. Now I always plan to make this for breakfast whenever eggplant was called for at dinner the previous night.

Serves 2 to 4

---

1 tbsp (15 mL) extra virgin olive oil

4 (½ inch [1 cm]) slices eggplant

½ tsp House Seasoning Blend (here)

1 clove garlic, thinly sliced

1 (14.5 oz [411 g]) can diced fire-roasted tomatoes

½ tsp dried basil

⅛ tsp kosher salt

Pinch of ground cinnamon

4 eggs

Chopped fresh Italian flat-leaf parsley, for garnish

Preheat the oven to 375°F (190°C) and also preheat a cast-iron or other oven-safe skillet over medium-high heat on the stovetop. Add the olive oil to the skillet.

Season both sides of the eggplant slices with the House Seasoning Blend. Sear the eggplant slices in the heated olive oil until golden brown on both sides. Remove from the pan and set aside. Replenish the fat as needed, then add the garlic slices and cook for just a few seconds. Add the tomatoes, basil, kosher salt and pinch of cinnamon.

Let the tomato sauce simmer for 3 to 5 minutes. Then nestle the seared eggplant slices into the sauce and top with an egg on each slice.

Pop the skillet in the oven and bake for 10 minutes for perfectly cooked egg whites with soft-cooked, creamy yolks. Serve directly from the skillet after garnishing with chopped fresh parsley.

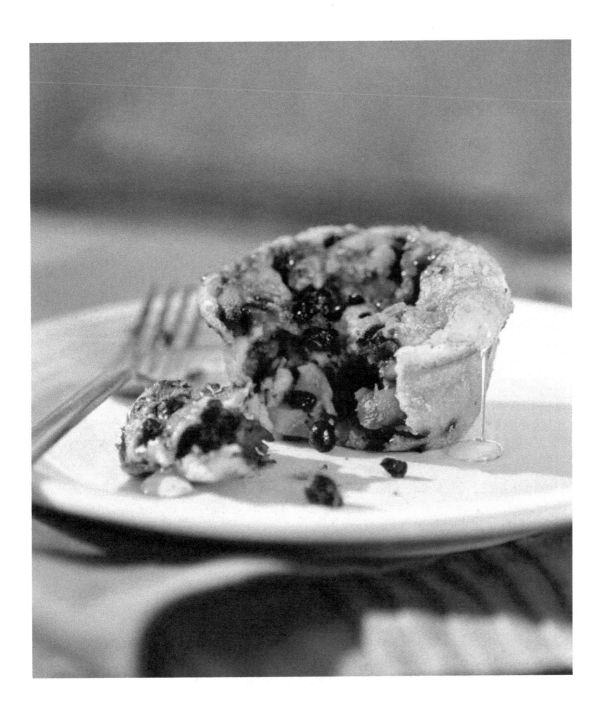

BLUEBERRY PEACH POPOVERS

Move over, cinnamon rolls. A new Saturday morning favorite is taking center stage: popovers. Naturally sweetened by fruit, these light and fluffy popovers are a treat your family will crave. We stopped going out for breakfast on Saturday mornings and now spend just a few dollars making this decadent meal at home. You'll see us eating these with a drizzle of honey on top and a few slices of bacon on the side!

Serves 6

3 tbsp (45 g) grass-fed butter or ghee

5 eggs

¾ cup (177 mL) almond milk

¼ cup (28 g) coconut flour

¼ cup (56 g) tapioca flour

¼ tsp salt

¼ tsp pure vanilla extract

¼ tsp ground cinnamon

1 (15 oz [411 g]) can peaches in juice

½ cup (115 g) frozen wild blueberries

Raw honey or organic maple syrup, for drizzling (optional)

Using a nonstick 6-cup popover pan, place equal amounts of the butter or ghee into the bottom of each cup. Place the pan in the oven and preheat to 425°F (218°C) so the pan warms and the butter melts. I like to set my popover pan on a baking sheet to make the transfers more secure and catch any spills while the popovers bake. Keep an eye on the butter to make sure you catch it before it burns.

Meanwhile, prepare the batter. Using a blender, food processor or stand mixer, combine the eggs, almond milk, flours, salt, vanilla and cinnamon and mix on high speed for 1 minute. It's fine if the coconut flour still appears a bit gritty.

The butter should be melted after only a few minutes. Remove the popover pan from the oven and place on the stovetop (or another heat-resistant surface). While the pan is still hot, place a single layer of peaches in the bottom of each cup (about 3 slices of canned peaches) and about a tablespoon (14 g) of frozen wild blueberries. Top each with a half cup of batter.

Bake for 18 to 22 minutes. The inside should just set and the outside will be golden brown. Allow to cool in the pan for 5 minutes, then use a large spoon to transfer to a serving dish and drizzle with raw honey or pure organic maple syrup, if desired. Serve warm.

TIP: Make 2 batches and save one for a quick breakfast during busy weekday mornings.

BRUSSELS SPROUT HASH

Community Supported Agriculture (CSA) boxes have become a popular source for local, organic produce. The weekly pick-up or delivery service is super convenient, local farms are supported and the vegetable selection is seasonal. Brussels sprouts seem to sneak their way into those weekly boxes fairly regularly, and I find that after a while some creativity in preparing them is necessary. So I started eating these little gems for breakfast! This hash makes for a quick and hearty start to the day.

Serves 2 to 3

---

2 cups (681 g) Brussels sprouts

½ small onion (about ¼ cup [40 g]), diced

3 slices bacon

Sea salt and black pepper, to taste

Additional bacon drippings or lard, if necessary

2 to 4 farm-fresh eggs

Prepare the fresh ingredients for the hash by trimming the core from the Brussels sprouts and slicing them in half—from the top of the sprout through the center core. Hang onto any leaves that fall away; they are welcome in the hash, too. And if the sprouts are a combination of large and small sizes, just halve the large ones and keep the small sprouts whole.

Dice the onion into small pieces. Hash is forgiving, so if the onion volume is more than a quarter cup (40 g), that's just fine. Grab about 3 bacon slices and stack them. Cut the bacon crosswise in about quarter-inch (6-mm) sections.

Heat a skillet over medium heat and add the bacon and onion. Cooking at this temperature will allow the bacon to render fat that should be sufficient for getting us through the hash. Cook until the onion has softened a bit and is slightly translucent, approximately 5 to 7 minutes. Now it's time to add the Brussels sprouts, a pinch of salt and a few grinds of black pepper. Season to your preference here.

The hash needs to be kept moving to prevent the onion from over-caramelizing and the sprouts from scorching. However, as welcome as loose leaves are in the hash, intact heads are preferred, so toss gently.

When the Brussels sprouts have softened to an al dente texture and taken on golden color, the bacon has crisped and the onion has caramelized (about 7 to 10 minutes), the hash is ready to transfer to a serving dish.

If the pan looks a little dry, replenish the fat with bacon drippings or lard, ideally. Other Paleo-friendly fats like tallow, duck fat, and olive, avocado or coconut oil will work as well. At medium heat, fry 2 to 4 eggs to your preference and lay them over the top of the hash for serving.

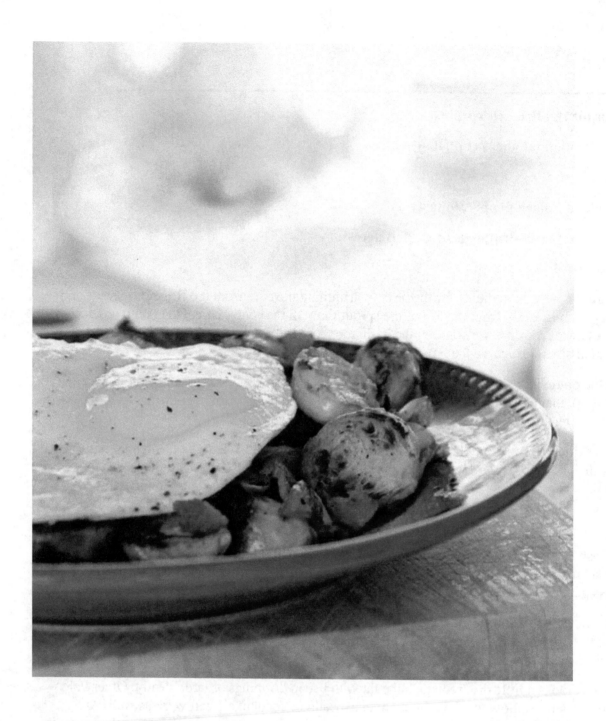

CARAMELIZED ONION FRITTATA

Frittatas are essentially a meat-and-veggie scramble that does not get mixed together. Instead, desired "fillings" are par-cooked, then topped with beaten eggs and cooked like a savory Dutch baby pancake. Budget-friendly and an excellent use for leftover protein and those last few veggies that need to be eaten, frittatas will be a mainstay in your Paleo kitchen. This particular recipe calls for eggs, onion and butter or ghee and feeds at least four people. It doesn't get much more affordable than that!

Serves 4 to 6

2 tbsp (30 mL) grass-fed butter or ghee

1 medium (about 3 inches [7.5 cm]) sweet onion

½ tsp kosher salt

8 eggs, beaten

¼ cup (40 g) cooked, chopped bacon (optional)

Black pepper, to taste

In a medium oven-safe skillet over medium heat, melt the butter or ghee.

To prepare the onion for caramelizing, remove both ends, slice in half from tip to root and then lay each half on the flat side. Work from end to end, cutting the onion into ⅛-inch (3-mm) strips. Do this for the entire onion. There should be about 2 ½ to 3 cups (300 g) of slices from a medium onion.

Drop the onion slices into the preheated pan. Add the kosher salt, cook and stir. Caramelizing onion is a slow process. Cooking too quickly will sauté the onion–delicious, but not what we're after for this recipe. Maintaining a moderate-to-low temperature and cooking over a longer period of time essentially melts or shrinks the onion. As it shrinks, it gradually becomes golden and somewhat on the sweet side. If, as you cook and stir the onion, it starts to scorch or brown unevenly, reduce the heat to medium-low, particularly if you are using a cast-iron skillet, which retains heat quite efficiently. Note, too, that the onion will require more stirring toward the end of the caramelization process than at the beginning.

Expect this to take approximately a half hour from start to finish. Meanwhile, beat the eggs together and set aside. When the onion is ready, reduce the heat to medium-low, if this wasn't done previously. Also, if you happen to have some leftover cooked bacon that you'd like to add to this frittata, now is the time to do that. Crumble a quarter cup (40 g) of bacon and mix it into the caramelized onion.

Pour in the beaten eggs and distribute the onion slices evenly throughout. This will ensure a balanced frittata when serving. Season to taste with black pepper.

Cook at medium-low, undisturbed, for about 4 minutes, or until the edges begin to pull away from the sides of the pan without breaking.

Transfer the frittata to the oven and turn the broiler to low to cook the top and finish setting the eggs. Place on the rack three rungs down from the top, or about 9 inches (23 cm) from the broiler. This should take approximately 5 to 6 minutes. The top of the frittata should be a deep orange to slightly golden, but not browned completely. The frittata should be somewhat firm to the touch and free of any pools of liquid from the beaten eggs.

Turn the oven off, return the pan to the stovetop, cover (foil is fine) and let rest for a minute or two. Resting allows the frittata to loosen from the pan, making service a breeze. Lift the frittata out of the pan and transfer to a cutting board. Slice into 6 wedges and serve.

CHICKEN FLORENTINE SKILLET

One of my keys to saving money is avoiding waste. After I roast a whole chicken or poach a few breasts for go-to protein during the week, I often have a small portion of meat left that needs a creative recipe to call home. This breakfast skillet does just that. Add some fresh spinach to savory onion and garlic, and you've got a hearty breakfast filled with flavor! Also, if you are on the Primal side of things, meaning you eat quality dairy products, top this dish with freshly grated Parmesan cheese or a few crumbles of feta. It's quite delicious.

Serves 2

---

1 tbsp (15 g) Paleo-friendly fat (lard, olive oil, grass-fed butter or ghee preferred)

1 cup (125 g) leftover shredded poached or roasted chicken (roughly 1 breast, shredded)

1 cup (38 g) packed, sliced organic baby spinach

½ cup (45 g) finely diced white or yellow onion (about 0.4 inch [1-cm] squares)

1 clove garlic, finely minced

4 eggs

Salt and pepper, to taste

Heat a seasoned cast-iron skillet or medium nonstick pan over medium heat. Add the selected Paleo-friendly fat to the pan and let it melt. I prefer grass-fed butter, ghee, olive oil or lard from pastured pigs in this recipe.

Add the chicken, spinach, onion and garlic to the pan. Cook and stir for 3 to 4 minutes, or until the onion becomes translucent, the garlic fragrant, the spinach wilted and the chicken browned slightly. Transfer the mixture to a bowl and set aside.

It may feel like a pain transferring everything to a bowl so the eggs cook separately, but it's the critical step for preparing a solid scramble. It makes all the difference between a proper-looking scramble and a bunch of eggs, meat and veggies that appear more like a broken frittata. Adding beaten eggs directly over the meat and veggies effectively acts like a sloppy, wet batter—yuck. We want stand-out pieces of shredded chicken, whole sautéed spinach and fluffy bites of scrambled egg here.

Return the pan to the heat and replenish some fat if the pan has dried out too much. Beat 4 eggs and pour into the hot pan. Season with salt and pepper, to taste. Gently shift the eggs as they cook. When the eggs are nearly cooked, but far too wet to call done, add the reserved chicken and vegetables back to the pan and gently fold to combine.

Cook for about 2 to 3 minutes, or until the eggs have lost their glossy sheen and are fully cooked. Serve immediately.

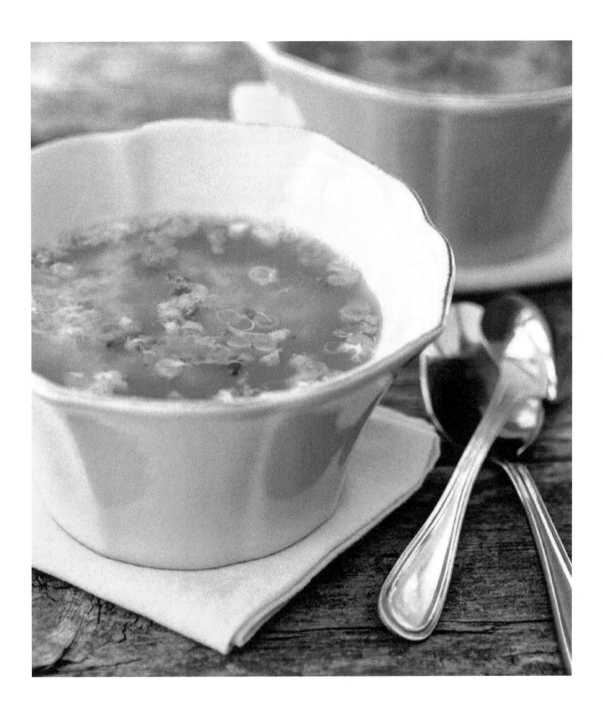

BREAKFAST SOUP

This wagon took me a hot minute to jump on to. Now that I have, I totally get what all the fuss was about. Starting the morning up with a hot cup of bone broth or a bowl of simple soup is an excellent way to wake up your digestive system. Sending nourishing, restorative foods into your body first thing will do so much to support gut health and boost immunity. I enjoy a bowl of this while I check emails and get myself organized for the day.

Serves 1

1 cup homemade bone broth (here)

1 egg, beaten

1 tbsp (15 g) cooked bacon crumbles

1 tsp (5 g) thinly sliced green onions

Salt and pepper, to taste

Hot sauce (optional)

Reheat a cup of homemade bone broth over medium heat until it bubbles slightly but does not boil. At that point, turn the burner off and stream in the beaten egg while gently stirring the broth to create somewhat of a whirlpool. The egg will scramble in the hot liquid and appear almost noodle like. Note: You may recognize this method. It's classic Asian egg drop soup!

When the egg has been added, pour into a bowl and top with the bacon crumbles and green onions. I like to add a little salt and pepper to balance the taste. Some days a couple splashes of hot sauce hit the spot! Do what sounds good to you.

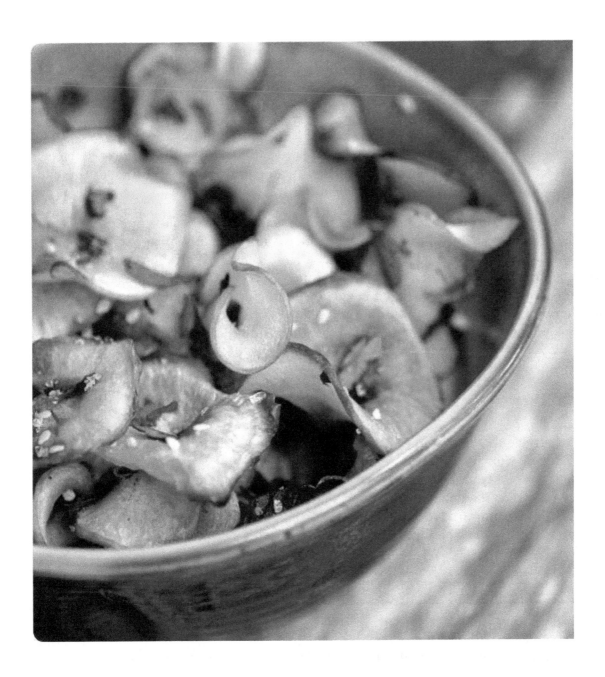

Confession: Before Paleo, I wasn't really a vegetable lover. Since a key principle in Paleo is a focus on nutrient-dense meals, I knew that I would need to up my game in the vegetable department.

In that spirit, I developed a challenge for myself and later extended it to my blog readers. Pick one vegetable a week that you aren't accustomed to eating or typically do not care for and prepare it in a recipe that is approachable and appealing. Ask your friends for recommendations or join a Paleo group on various social media platforms. People love to share ideas for healthy recipes!

Through this challenge I confirmed that eggplant still isn't high on my list and, if I'm being honest, I really don't care for asparagus. But I also discovered that my kids absolutely love parsnips, kale, carrots, broccoli, cauliflower, green beans and bell peppers. We eat a lot of Brussels sprouts, too. And we almost never eat traditional salads—these are all veggie dishes independently prepared, like the recipes you'll find in the following chapter, or are a part of the one-dish meals you'll find in the protein chapters.

Another way to get more vegetables into your diet is to change up the way they are prepared by looking into other cooking methods. For example, I don't love Swiss chard on its own or the texture when sautéed, but I can't get enough of crispy, spicy Charps (here). Changing the way the vegetable was prepared made it a new favorite!

Playing around with textures and methods is also a great way to take advantage of a sale. When you come across a good deal on produce, such as maybe a buy-one-get-one-free for organic cauliflower, stock up and use this tactic. A simple head of cauliflower can be mashed for faux mashed potatoes, transformed into Moroccan Cauli-Rice (here) for an exotic grain-free side dish or roasted on the grill with daring spices like cacao and chili powder (here) to give that boring cauliflower a serious Cinderella story. That's three very different tastes and textures using one basic vegetable. And that's exactly how I stretch a buck when it comes to vegetables.

CHARPS

By now I'm sure you've made your share of kale chips, so let me introduce you to Charps (Chard + Chips = Charps). They're the ideal nutrient-dense Paleo snack when you're craving something salty and crunchy. Next time you reach for that bunch of kale, stop and move a few veggies to the left or right to find some chard instead. Chard has a nuttier, more earthy flavor compared to kale and is significantly higher in iron, a vital mineral. And a bonus? It's usually a smidge cheaper.

Serves 2

---

1 bunch organic chard

1 tbsp (15 g) Paleo-friendly fat, melted (I prefer ghee, grass-fed butter or avocado oil)

1 tsp (5 g) salt-free seasoning blend (I recommend House Seasoning Blend, here)

Sea salt, to taste

Preheat the oven to 300°F (149°C).

Wash and thoroughly, but gently, dry the chard. Tear the leaves into 2- to 3-inch (5-to 7-cm) segments, or your desired "chip" size. Be sure to trim and discard the stems because they maintain more moisture than the leaves and throw off cook times.

In a large bowl, toss the chard leaf segments with the melted fat. Sprinkle in the seasoning blend and toss to evenly coat the leaves.

In a single layer, place the chard on a nonstick baking surface such as a baking sheet lined with parchment or a silicone mat. Bake for 15 to 17 minutes.

Remove from the oven, transfer to a serving dish and toss quickly with finer-grain sea salt while still hot. Let cool and crunch away!

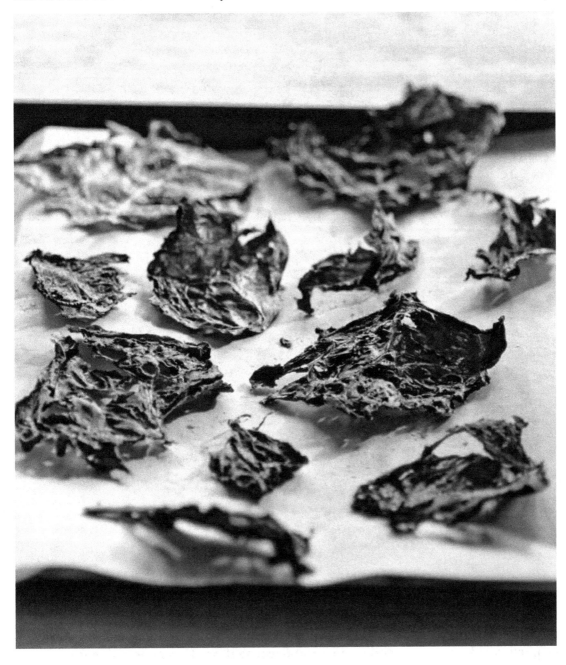

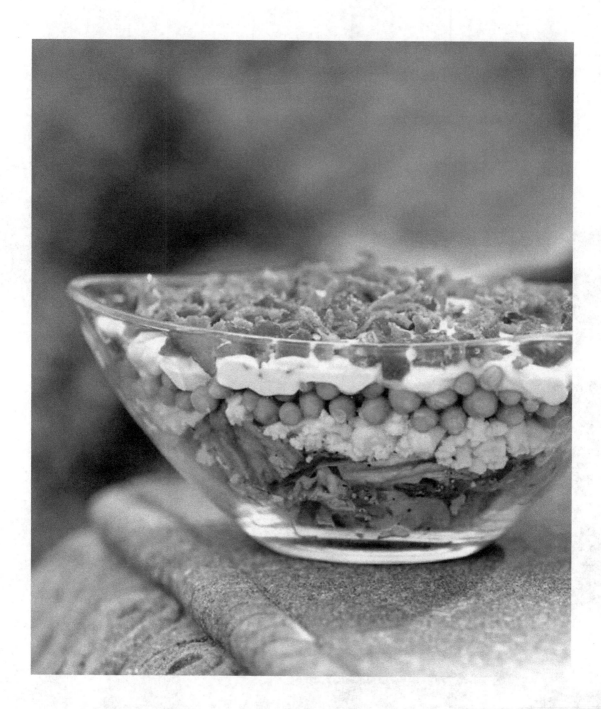

OVERNIGHT SALAD

This salad was a favorite of mine growing up. My grandmother would make it for family gatherings, particularly for my birthday (in July) because it went great as a side for barbecuing burgers and dogs. Now my own family gets to enjoy it thanks to homemade mayo, and I think it's even better than the original!

Serves 6 to 8

½ head organic green or red leaf lettuce

Black pepper, to taste

6 hard-cooked eggs, peeled and chopped

2 cups (300 g) peas (thawed, if frozen; drained, if canned)

1 cup (237 mL) Homemade Mayonnaise (here)

½ tsp nutritional yeast (optional)

1 cup (175 g) chopped, cooked bacon

This is a layered salad that actually sets—you guessed it—overnight. It's served chilled and is nearly a complete meal on its own. Here's how you make it:

Clean and dry the lettuce leaves. Chop, slice or tear into a good size for salad.

Layer the salad in a deep 8-inch by 11-inch (20-cm by 28-cm) casserole dish, preferably with a lid, in this order:

Lettuce

A few grinds of black pepper, to taste

Chopped hard-cooked eggs

Peas

Mayo, spread evenly across the top

Nutritional yeast, if you are using[*]

Bacon bits

*The nutritional yeast replaces cheese in the original recipe, but it's not a required ingredient. I buy mine bulk at my local health food store and find it affordable.

Cover and store in the refrigerator overnight or for at least a few hours. Serve chilled.

MUSHROOM DIAVOLO

Grilling a steak? You've gotta pair it with Mushroom Diavolo! "Diavolo" comes from the Italian word devil and is used as a culinary term to connote spicy. It's more of an Italian-American thing, but that makes no difference to me. Spicy, buttery, garlicky mushrooms are what I'm after, and once you taste these, you'll know why I'm hooked.

Serves 2

---

8 oz (230 g) button mushrooms

2 cloves garlic

¼ cup (55 g) grass-fed butter, plus another tbsp (15 g) of lard or Paleo-friendly fat

¼ tsp red-pepper flakes Pinch of coarse sea salt

Chopped fresh Italian flat-leaf parsley, for garnish (optional)

Heat a cast-iron skillet over medium heat.

Clean the mushrooms by wiping with the grain using a dry towel, basically from the top toward the stem. Mushrooms are super absorbent and will soak up anything they come in contact with. In order to avoid soggy 'shrooms, use a dry towel to remove any dirt still stuck to them.

Trim the dry, discolored portion of the stem and slice the mushroom in half, from top to stem.

Slice the garlic as thin as you're able. I prefer sliced to minced for this recipe for textural reasons, but if you just can't bring yourself to practice those knife skills, by all means, mince away.

Melt the quarter cup (55 g) butter in the skillet, add the mushrooms and carefully toss to coat. Cook until the butter has evenly glazed the mushrooms and they've begun to take on some color, about 4 minutes. Add the garlic and red-pepper flakes. Be sure to keep this moving as it cooks. Garlic burns easily and will become bitter. Slices help to stave it off, but it's no guarantee. Plus, continually tossing the mushrooms in the fat, garlic and pepper flakes yields a more balanced flavor since they will be more evenly coated in all those delicious, bold spices.

Should the pan start to look a bit dry, add another tablespoon (15 g) of fat. Remember that those mushrooms have absorbed a fair amount of fat at this point, so the need to replenish is quite likely. I prefer to use another fat to vary the flavor. Butter with a boost of fresh lard did the trick for me. However, tallow, duck fat or even coconut oil would be suitable. Be sure to add the fat directly to the bottom of the pan and not on top of any mushrooms, or you'll turn those little guys into oil slicks.

When the mushrooms have become golden and the garlic has crisped without becoming burnt, it's time to remove them from the heat, transfer to a serving dish and sprinkle on a pinch of coarse sea salt. Have some flat-leaf parsley on hand? Chop up a few sprigs and use it as a garnish. Serve hot.

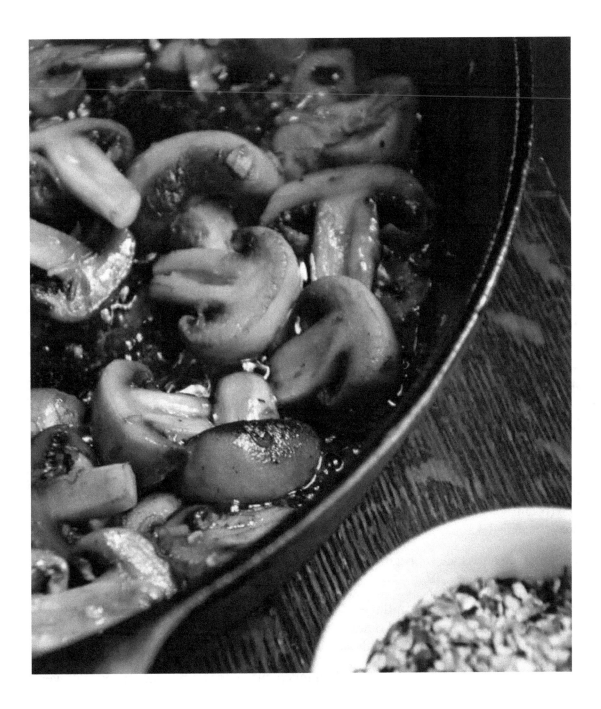

BOLLYWOOD SLAW

I love traditional coleslaw, but sometimes even the classics need a boost of flavor from time to time. In this case, coleslaw is getting a complete face-lift—Indian style! Transform bland coleslaw into something exotic with a homemade curry aioli, crisp apple and sweet raisins. Just look what you can create with a few pantry spices and two low-cost produce items!

Serves 4 to 6

Half of 1 organic cabbage (about 6 cups [2 kg] shredded)

1 organic green apple

1 organic red apple

½ cup (75 g) golden raisins

½ cup (118 mL) Homemade Mayonnaise (here)

½ tsp garlic powder

½ tsp ground turmeric

1 tsp (5 g) curry powder

¼ cup (60 mL) unflavored kombucha tea or fresh organic apple juice

Chopped fresh cilantro, for garnish (optional)

Split a head of cabbage in half from the top of the head through the center of the core. Flip it flat side down and halve it again, splitting down the center of the core. Use a sharp knife and a steady hand to shred the cabbage from the top of the head down through the wedge until you reach the core, which can be discarded. Do this for both wedges; half of a head of cabbage should yield around 6 cups (2 kg) of thin shreds.

Move to the apples next. I prefer to keep the peels on in this recipe. Julienne both apples. Do this by slicing alongside the core, not through it. Continue slicing to the side of the core, cutting the apple into sections and removing the core (which gets discarded). Slice each apple segment into quarter-inch (6-mm) pieces. Next, stack a few slices on top of each other and slice through them again to create matchsticks.

In a large mixing bowl, toss the cabbage, apples and raisins.

Separately whip up the curry aioli. In a small mixing bowl, combine the mayo with the garlic powder, turmeric, curry powder and unflavored kombucha tea. Home-brewed kombucha is the most cost-effective option for sourcing kombucha. However, if this isn't an option and you must substitute, use some organic apple juice with no added sugar instead.

When the curry aioli is well combined and evenly thinned out by the kombucha tea, pour it over the slaw and toss to combine.

It's best to cover the slaw and allow it to chill in the refrigerator for 1 to 2 hours before serving. Mix it once more and top with chopped fresh cilantro when the time comes to set it on your table—dining room or picnic alike.

PAN-ROASTED CAULIFLOWER AND ZUCCHINI

I like to make this easy side dish when zucchini is at the height of the season in late summer. It seems gardens everywhere are overflowing with them. Many recipes seek to manipulate both of these vegetables in Paleo since they do make convenient grain-free

substitutes (including several recipes in this book). However, let's not forget how great they can be when prepared in their original forms as well.

Serves 4

¼ cup (55 g) coconut oil

Half of 1 head cauliflower, cut into florets

2 zucchini, cut into large dice

2 cloves garlic, minced

½ tsp dried Italian seasoning

¼ tsp onion powder

¼ tsp sea salt

Pinch of red-pepper flakes

Chopped fresh Italian flat-leaf parsley, for garnish

In a large pan or skillet, melt the coconut oil over medium-high heat. Once the oil is hot (is glossy and moves easily across the pan when tilted from side to side), add the cauliflower and cook, stirring often, for 3 to 5 minutes, or until it takes on a little color. Cauliflower takes longer to cook than zucchini, so it needs the head start.

Next add the zucchini, garlic and spices. Toss to bring everything together and continue to cook for 7 minutes or so, stirring often.

Notice the progression of the garlic as the dish cooks. As you become more familiar with cooking with whole foods, learn to use your sense of smell as well as sight to determine the doneness of a dish. For example, with garlic it's easy to identify when it is raw (pungent), then warmed (sweet) and then suddenly burnt (bitter). Cooked garlic is ideal when in the sweet stage.

Cook the vegetables until the cauliflower has a visible golden crust, the zucchini is softened and the garlic is sweetly fragrant and no longer pungent; this should take about 10 to 12 minutes from start to finish. Transfer to a serving dish and top with some fresh chopped Italian flat-leaf parsley. Serve warm.

KOHLRABI "PAPADUM" CHIPS

These chips remind me of the crisp wafer bread at Indian restaurants called papadum. Though papadums are generally made from a lentil flour dough and fried, once these kohlrabi chips are seasoned with sesame seeds and fresh parsley, the taste brings me back to my favorite little neighborhood Indian joint, snacking on papadum and raita on a rainy Pacific Northwest day. Pick up a kohlrabi for a few cents and give this one a try!

Serves 2

---

1 large kohlrabi

1 tbsp (15 g) coconut oil

Pinch of coarse-grain sea salt

1 tbsp (3 g) chopped fresh flat-leaf parsley

½ tsp toasted sesame seeds

Trim the leaves and stems as close to the kohlrabi bulb as possible and scrub it well under running water.

Set a mandoline to the thinnest setting and slice the unpeeled kohlrabi into "chips."

Lay the slices in a single layer on an aerated baking sheet. A solid baking sheet can be used as well, but it should be lined with parchment or another nonstick surface.

Place in the oven and heat to 200°F (94°C). Bake for 1 hour on the aerated pan or 1 ½ hours on the solid baking sheet. Turn the slices once about halfway through. Remove the cooked slices from the baking sheet and set out to cool on a clean, dry surface.

In a small high-sided pan over medium-high heat, warm the coconut oil. Keep some extra on hand just in case the pan starts to dry out as the kohlrabi are fried.

Working 1 chip at a time, use a pair of tongs to hold on to a small edge of the chip. Fry each side for no more than 3 seconds. In fact, count "1, 2, 3, flip" and then "1, 2, done." They really fry that fast. Transfer to a dish lined with a disposable towel to absorb excess oil and hold. Repeat until all of the chips are fried.

Season the kohlrabi chips with a pinch of sea salt, the chopped parsley and a sprinkle of toasted sesame seeds.

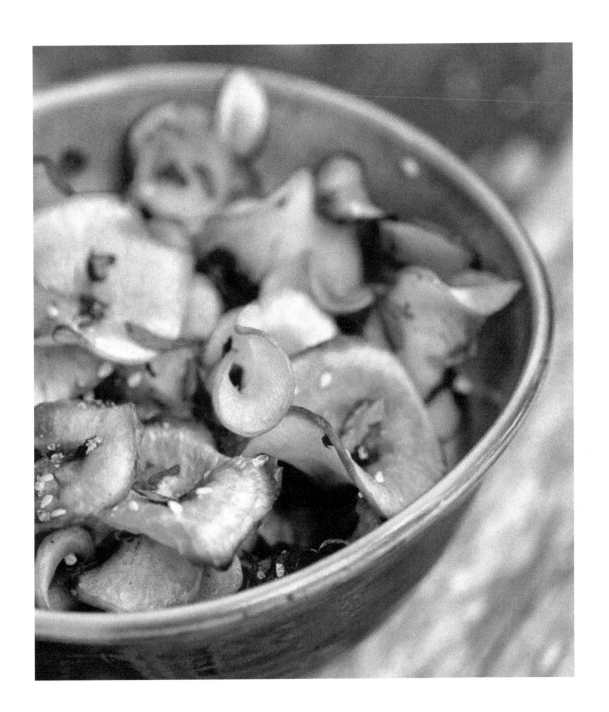

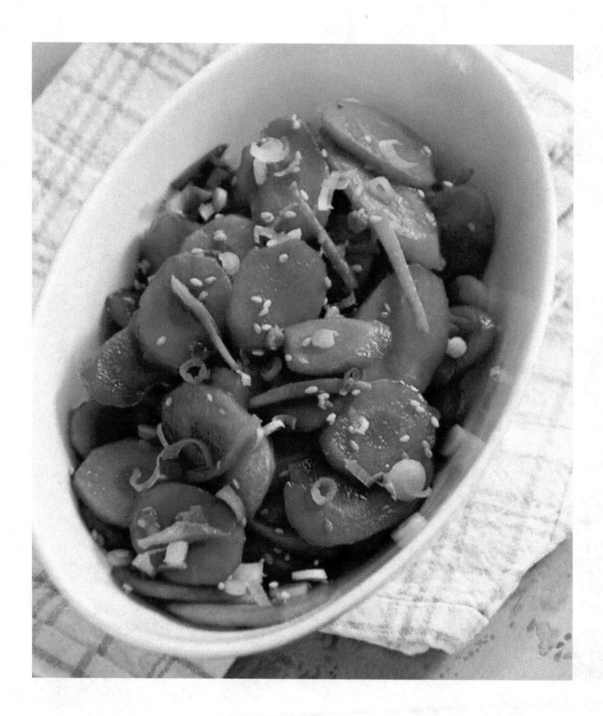

GINGER CARROTS

I like to keep a bottle of coconut aminos in my refrigerator since it makes an excellent soy-free, gluten-free substitute for soy sauce. While it is a bit more per ounce than regular soy sauce, I can stretch my purchase by using just a little bit to create an easy Asian glaze over sautéed organic carrots. This is an easy side dish that takes minutes to prepare and partners well with Asian-Style Prawns (here), Stupid Easy Asian Beef (here) or Ground Beef Stir-Fry with Wilted Cabbage (here) to round off an ethnic Paleo feast.

Serves 2 or 3

1 lb (454 g) organic carrots

1 inch (2.5 cm) gingerroot

Paleo-friendly fat, such as lard, tallow, duck fat, coconut oil or avocado oil

¼ tsp kosher salt

¼ cup (60 mL) coconut aminos

1 tbsp (5 g) thinly sliced green onions

½ tsp toasted sesame seeds

½ tsp chia seeds (optional)

Peel the carrots, remove the tops (if applicable) and slice diagonally about ⅛-inch (3-mm) thick. Peel the gingerroot and slice into matchsticks.

Heat a heavy-bottomed pan over medium heat and melt a few teaspoons (10 g) of coconut oil (or preferred Paleo-friendly fat).

Drop the carrots, ginger and kosher salt into the hot pan. Cook and stir until the carrots are just tender, about 5 to 7 minutes.

Add the coconut aminos and deglaze the pan by scraping up the browned bits off the bottom as the coconut aminos cook out. Simmer for about 3 to 4 minutes to reduce the coconut aminos into a light glaze before transferring to a serving dish.

Once carrots are plated, sprinkle on the green onions, toasted sesame seeds and chia seeds for garnish. Serve hot.

SPICY BEET SALAD

Grocers are getting wise to the demand for organic, non-GMO produce and making it easier than ever to find quality vegetables and fruit. I find ready-to-eat beets for a very good price at my local wholesale grocery retailer and skip the process of preparing them myself. Remember your time is valuable, too, so when you get a chance to save some, take it! And if your local grocery store doesn't carry ready-to-eat beets, don't worry. They are simple enough to prepare. (See below for a quick How-To.)

Serves 4

½ cup (118 mL) Homemade Mayonnaise (here)

2 tbsp (30 g) freshly grated horseradish root (or 1 tsp [5 mL] prepared horseradish sauce, see below)

1 tsp (5 g) chopped fresh rosemary

1 tsp (5 mL) apple cider vinegar

¼ tsp kosher salt

2 tbsp (5 g) chopped fresh flat-leaf parsley

A few grinds of black pepper

4 ready-to-eat organic, non-GMO beets (about 2 cups [400 g])

In a medium bowl, combine the mayonnaise with all of the remaining ingredients, except for the beets. When it comes to the horseradish root, a microplane or zesting tool is ideal. Larger shavings won't incorporate into the dressing properly, so be sure to take the time to finely grate the root after peeling the section of the root that will be grated. Once the ingredients are well mixed, move to slicing the beets.

Cut the beets into ⅛-inch-thick (3-mm-thick) slices. You should have enough to yield approximately 2 cups (400 g). Add directly to the dressing and carefully combine to fully coat the beets. If the beets have been freshly roasted, ensure that they have cooled completely before adding them to the dressing or the texture will change from the heat.

This salad is delicious cold, so allow it to chill in the refrigerator for an hour or so, covered, before serving. Additional chopped flat-leaf parsley for garnish is a nice touch, if you'd like.

Not able to find ready-to-eat beets? They're easy to do yourself. Preheat the oven to 400°F (204°C). Trim the greens from 4 beets and roast them in the oven for about 40 minutes. When they're done, allow a few minutes for cooling. When you're able to comfortably handle the beets, peel them and slice ⅛-inch (3-mm) thick. Completely cool the beets before incorporating with the dressing, so the mayo doesn't warm and change texture.

Why fresh horseradish? The processed spreads have far too many additives for my liking. Like mayonnaise, this is one sauce that should really be made from scratch.

Peel a 5- to 6-inch (8- to 15-cm) horseradish root with a vegetable peeler and chop it into pieces.

Add the pieces to a food processor plus 2 or 3 tablespoons (30 to 45 mL) of water and puree. Stand back! Horseradish is intense and can irritate your eyes and nose. Turn the food processor off, and add a pinch of sea salt and about a tablespoon (15 mL) of white vinegar. Scrape down the sides with a rubber spatula, then pulse a few more times to incorporate the salt and vinegar.

Transfer to a glass jar with a tight-fitting lid and refrigerate. This should keep for just under a month, so be sure to note the date on the jar.

Should you decide to process your horseradish root first and then make Spicy Beet Salad, add just a teaspoon (5 mL) to the dressing. The horseradish concentrates when broken down, and a little will go a long way.

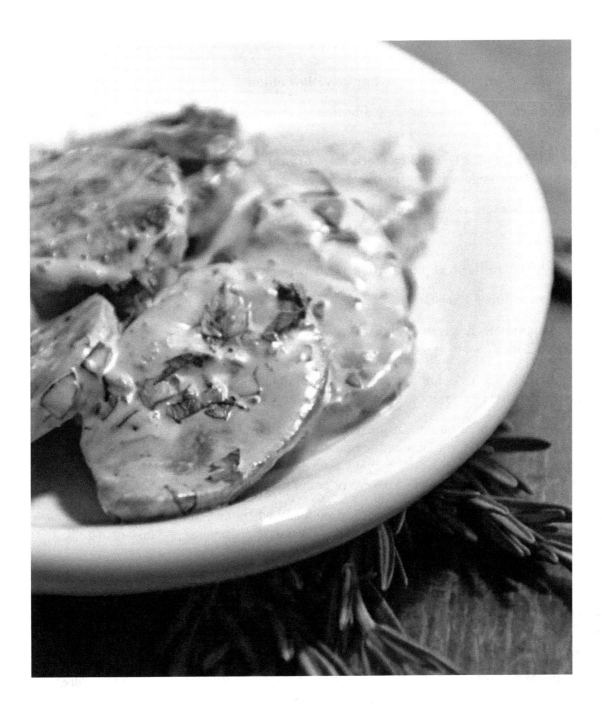

ROASTED CARROT SOUP

The ideal soup for fall, roasted carrots and onion pureed together create a simple yet rich soup that perfectly complements the changing weather outside. Serve this soup alongside a Roasted French Countryside Chicken (here) and Hard Cider Sprouts (here) for a memorable, yet affordable, family-style Paleo meal.

Serves 4 to 6

2 lb (908 g) organic carrots

1 small (2 inches [5 cm] in diameter) white or yellow onion

1 tbsp (15 g) Paleo-friendly fat (grass-fed butter, ghee or lard work particularly well with this soup)

4 to 5 cups (948 mL to 1.2 L) chicken stock from organic, free-range chickens (use vegetable stock for a vegetarian option)

1 batch Autumn Seasoning Blend (here)

1 tsp (5 g) sea salt

Chopped fresh Italian flat-leaf parsley, for garnish

Preheat the oven to 400°F (204°C).

Peel the carrots, trim off the greens and discard. Slice the carrots lengthwise in half first, then chop into about 2-inch (5-cm) chunks. Place in a medium mixing bowl.

Peel and quarter the onion. Add it to the carrots. Melt the fat of your choice and pour it over the carrots and onion. Toss to evenly coat.

Arrange the vegetables on a parchment-lined baking sheet large enough to allow a couple inches (several centimeters) of space in between segments. In order to properly roast the vegetables, the pan must not be overcrowded. Overcrowding would essentially bake the carrots and onion, yielding a much different flavor than what we're going for here.

Roast the vegetables for 30 to 35 minutes. They are ready when the carrots are completely cooked through and both the carrots and onion have begun to caramelize and take on a golden brown color, particularly on the side that rested on the parchment.

Transfer the vegetables directly to a food processor or high-capacity blender. Puree immediately.

As the vegetables puree, pour in the chicken stock and add the Autumn Seasoning Blend and salt. (For a thicker soup, use only 4 cups [948 mL] of the stock.) Continue to puree until a smooth texture is achieved.

Serve immediately. Chopped fresh flat-leaf parsley makes a wonderful garnish, if you desire.

PUNJABI CABBAGE

This is a simplified version of the traditional dish meant to ease the pressure off your wallet and your spice cabinet. The heart of the recipe is still intact—onion, garlic, ginger, cabbage and those familiar exotic flavors, thanks to Indian Seasoning Blend. Because this dish is quite bold, I recommend pairing it with simple grilled or roasted chicken.

Serves 4

1 tbsp (15 g) coconut oil (ghee could be substituted)

1 medium yellow onion, diced

3 cloves garlic, minced

Half of 1 head organic cabbage, chopped

½ inch (1 cm) gingerroot, finely diced

1 batch Indian Seasoning Blend (here)

½ tsp kosher salt

⅛ tsp crushed red-pepper flakes

Heat a large skillet over medium-high heat and melt the coconut oil. When the oil is hot (is glossy and moves easily when the pan is tilted from side to side), add the onion, ginger and garlic. Cook and stir occasionally for 8 to 9 minutes, or until just starting to brown.

Add the chopped cabbage and all of the spices to the onion mixture and combine well. Cook and stir for 10 to 12 minutes, or until the cabbage reaches a texture that you prefer. I like a slight al dente texture, which is accomplished after 10 minutes or so.

Transfer to a serving dish and enjoy!

APPLE BUTTERNUT HASH

This recipe is a great alternative to sweet potato hash. I find that I eat sweet potatoes a lot with lunch and dinner, so when it comes to breakfast, I like to play with other options. Butternut squash pairs very well with apples, especially the sweet ones like Honeycrisp, and together along with Breakfast Seasoning Blend (here), they create a sweet and savory breakfast hash that tastes like it was borrowed from a Thanksgiving pie.

Serves 2 to 3

1 ½ to 2 lb (683 to 908 g) butternut squash

1 large sweet apple, such as Honeycrisp

2 tbsp (30 g) grass-fed butter or ghee

1 batch Breakfast Seasoning Blend (here)

½ tsp kosher salt

¼ cup (25 g) chopped walnuts (optional)

Start by preparing the butternut squash. Trim off each end and use a vegetable peeler to remove the tough peel. Slice in half lengthwise down the center and use a spoon to scrape out the seeds and pulp. Cut the squash into bite-size cubes.

Prepare the apple by slicing in half (from stem to base) just to the right of the core; don't slice through the core, slice alongside it. Then lay the apple cut side down and slice alongside the core again. Repeat until the core is removed and the apple is cut into (uneven) sections. Cut the apple sections into bite-size pieces, the same size as the squash. It's okay to leave the peel on the apple; lots of nutrients are in the peel, let's eat that.

Heat a pan over medium heat and melt the butter or ghee. Add the cubed squash next and toss to coat in the melted butter/ghee. Continue to stir occasionally as the squash cooks for 10 to 12 minutes. The mixture will appear quite buttery, and that's okay. There's enough fat to coat the apples and absorb the spices that are coming up.

Add the cubed apple to the squash as well as the Breakfast Seasoning Blend and kosher salt. Thoroughly combine all of the ingredients so the spices are evenly distributed and continue to cook for another 10 to 12 minutes, stirring occasionally.

When the squash and apple have softened and a nice glaze has formed, transfer to a serving dish. If desired, sprinkle chopped walnuts over the top of the hash.

CHINESE-STYLE BROCCOLINI

Growing up in a Chinese home, we ate something similar to this often. This recipe simplifies what I grew up eating, plus substitutes healthier ingredients such as coconut aminos for traditional soy sauce and coconut oil for vegetable oil. Once your pantry is converted to a Paleo-one, you'll just need to pick up some Broccolini to complete this quick side dish.

Serves 2 to 4

---

1 tbsp (15 g) coconut oil

8 oz Broccolini (about 1 ½ cups [225 g])

1 inch (2.5 cm) gingerroot, peeled and cut into matchsticks

2 cloves garlic, chopped

¼ cup (60 mL) coconut aminos

Toasted sesame and chia seeds, for garnish (optional)

Heat a heavy-bottomed pan over medium-high heat and melt the coconut oil. Trim about a half inch (1 cm) or so from the Broccolini stems.

Place the Broccolini in the pan and let it brown up—don't move it around right away! A slight char is good. Give it a minute or 2, then add the ginger and garlic and toss to combine.

Reduce the heat to medium and cook for 3 to 5 minutes. Add the coconut aminos to deglaze the pan. The aminos will reduce quickly, so keep the Broccolini (but especially the garlic) moving at this point. Try to coat the Broccolini as evenly as possible with the light glaze that's developing.

Remove from the heat, transfer to a serving dish and garnish with sesame and chia seeds, if desired. I like the nod of nutrients the chia seeds offer, and I like the tan and black contrast between the two seeds, but that part is optional.

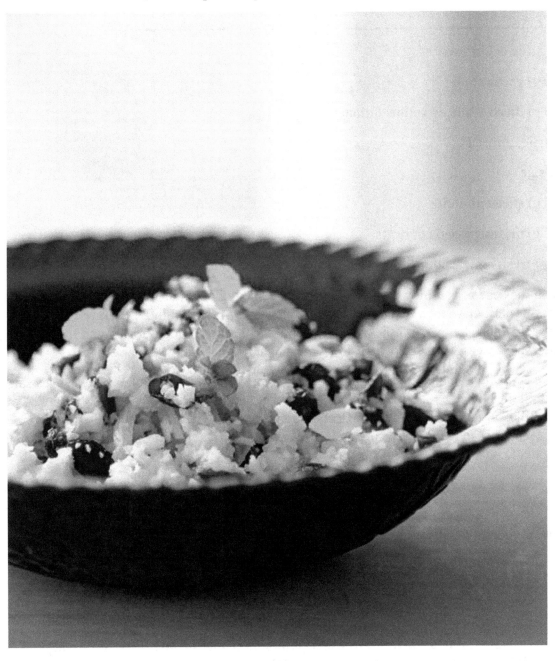

MOROCCAN CAULI-RICE

Once you get the hang of making rice out of cauliflower, the sky's the limit when it comes to flavor combinations. I like this recipe because it feels uber-gourmet without the costly ingredients. Other popular options include cilantro-lime; Spanish Rice-style with taco seasoning, tomatoes and green onions; and even shredded carrots, bacon and scrambled eggs with coconut aminos for a Paleo Fried Rice. Get familiar with the cauliflower rice method and have fun experimenting in the kitchen with new ideas!

Serves 4 to 6

---

1 head organic cauliflower

2 tbsp (30 g) coconut oil

½ cup (75 g) diced white or yellow onion

1 clove garlic, minced

½ tsp sea salt

2 tbsp (15 g) sliced almonds

2 tbsp (20 g) organic dried currants

1 tbsp (3 g) fresh mint, chopped or torn

Break down the head of cauliflower into large florets. Working in batches, pulse the florets in a food processor until they reach a rice-like texture. Personally, I don't mind the larger stem pieces that don't seem to break down as quickly. I know this is cauliflower and I don't mind the size discrepancies. Set the riced cauliflower aside; you should have about 4 cups (1 L).

Heat a large skillet over medium heat and melt the coconut oil. Add the onion, garlic and sea salt and cook until the onion has softened and become somewhat translucent, about 6 to 8 minutes. Add the cauliflower to the pan and continue cooking for another 10 to 15 minutes. The cauliflower will need to release moisture and soften a bit. Remove the cauliflower from the heat before it starts to brown.

When the cauli-rice is tender, add the almonds, dried currants and fresh mint. Stir together and let cook for just 3 to 5 minutes more.

Transfer to a serving bowl and garnish with additional sliced mint (and/or sliced almonds, too, if you like).

SWEET POTATO TATER TOTS

I'd like to say that I came up with these sweet potato tater tots for my kids, but we all know the truth. Adults love these just as much as kids do! Tater Tots are an irresistible crunchy

side dish, which can actually be made Paleo-friendly thanks to a couple of sweet potatoes—not yams—and some good-quality oil for frying.

Serves 4 to 6

---

2 to 2 ½ lb (908 g to 1.1 kg) yellow sweet potatoes (not yams)

½ cup (118 mL) Paleo-friendly fat (I prefer lard, duck fat, avocado oil or coconut oil)

Pinch of salt (I like coarse-grain Celtic sea salt)

Preheat the oven to 400°F (204°C). Wash the sweet potatoes and poke a few times with a fork. Place the sweet potatoes on a baking sheet lined with parchment paper and bake for 35 to 40 minutes. Carefully remove from the oven and set aside to cool to room temperature. This will take a few hours, so plan ahead.

When the potatoes are cool enough to handle, remove the skin. It should easily slide off when you drag the back of a butter knife across it. Discard the peels.

Using a box grater, shred the sweet potatoes. The potatoes should be somewhat sticky from having the intrinsic sugars activated from the baking. In fact, it's the natural sugars from the sweet potatoes that act as the binder for the tot.

Use a tablespoon or something comparable to scoop out spoonfuls of shredded potato. Working one at a time, roll the potatoes back and forth in the palm of your hand a few times, then squish the ends flat to create the classic Tater Tot shape. Continue working until all of the potato is used up.

Now move to frying the newly formed tots. I like to use an 8-inch (20-cm) cast-iron skillet because it is narrow with high sides. This means less oil is needed, which saves money. There is some flexibility on which Paleo-friendly oil to select, but in general animal-based fats will yield a better flavor, so my vote is for lard from pastured pigs or duck fat. In the event you don't have these on hand, avocado oil works great—as does coconut oil. Avoid oils with low smoke points like olive or bacon drippings. They won't fry properly.

Melt or heat your chosen fat in a small, high-sided pan at just shy of high heat. Don't max out your dial, but get it pretty close.

When the oil is hot, fry 5 or 6 tots at a time, working in batches. Frying only a few at a time will keep the oil temperature stable. This means the tots will have a crispy outside and a creamy inside.

Each side requires only about a minute or so to brown, so keep a close eye on the tots and always be ready to turn and/or remove them. The end caps don't generally need frying since the oil level is likely high enough to brown the edges.

Once the Tater Tots are golden brown, remove them from the oil and transfer to a surface lined with paper towels to drain. Repeat until all of the tots are cooked.

Season with salt (I like coarse-grain Celtic sea salt on these) and maybe a sprinkling of House Seasoning Blend (here) for an extra kick. Serve with your favorite Paleo dipping sauce or use these to make Paleo Hotdish (here)—more commonly known as Tater Tot Casserole.

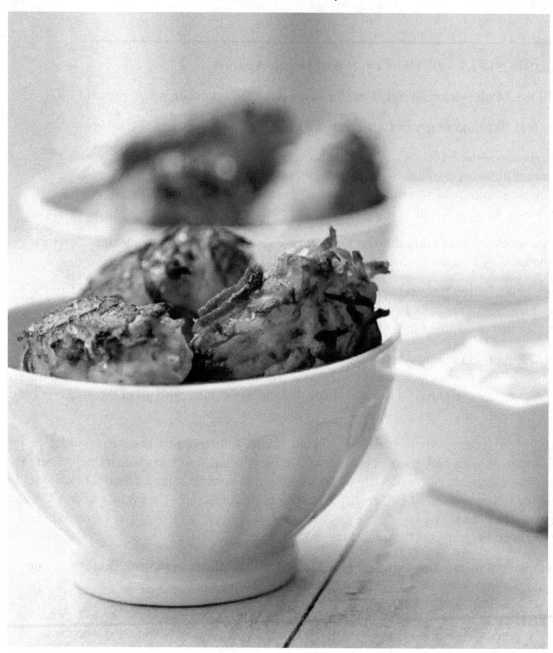

EASY AVOCADO LIME SALAD

I truly believe that Paleo food is simple food. It's easy to be impressed by the fancy recipes creative cooks can put together using basic meat, vegetables, fruits, nuts and seeds. I'm proud to be one of those people. However, this recipe represents real life. Real life is filled with sliced veggies, scrambled eggs, a handful of nuts and easy grilled meats. In that spirit,

this avocado recipe was born. I eat this at least once a week and love it as a side to Chicken and Chorizo Meatballs (here).

Serves 2

---

1 avocado

1 lime

¼ cup (7 g) fresh chopped cilantro

½ tsp coarse-grain sea salt

Pinch of crushed red-pepper flakes, a few jalapeño slices or a few dashes of hot sauce

Slice the avocado in half lengthwise (from stem to base), circling the knife around the pit. Twist both hemispheres to release. To remove the pit, hold the half securely in one hand and with the other, whack the knife blade into the pit and give the knife a little twist. The pit should pop right out. Set down the avocado and grab a kitchen towel. Grip the pit with the towel and pull the pit off the knife blade, carefully.

Without breaking through the peel, cut the flesh of the avocado into slices about a half inch (1 cm) thick or so. Then use a spoon to scoop the avocado slices out of the shell by running the spoon between the flesh of the avocado and the peel. Let the slices fall out right onto your plate or serving dish. Repeat with the other avocado half for the second serving.

Slice the lime in half and squeeze the fresh juice on the avocado; one half for each serving.

Sprinkle the avocado with the cilantro and sea salt. If you'd like to add some heat to this dish, top with a pinch of crushed red-pepper flakes, some jalapeño slices or even just a few dashes of hot sauce, whatever sounds good to you.

BOMBAY PARSNIP AND CARROT FRIES

Jazz up basic roasted root veggies with exotic Indian spices. Use whatever Paleo-friendly fat you have on hand and a sprinkle of something different from your spice cabinet with basic carrots and parsnips. Super simple, a lot of flavor and very easy on the wallet.

Serves 4

---

1 parsnip

4 organic carrots

1 tsp (5 g) Indian Seasoning Blend (here)

1 tbsp (15 g) Paleo-friendly fat, melted (coconut oil, avocado oil and ghee work well)

Coarse sea salt

Preheat the oven to 425°F (218°C).

Peel the parsnip and carrots and cut into steak fries. Try your best to make them as uniform as possible so they will cook evenly. Place in a large bowl.

If you don't already have a batch of Indian Seasoning Blend (here) on hand, mix that up now. We'll need a teaspoon (5 g) for seasoning the carrots and parsnips.

Melt your selected Paleo-friendly fat, add it to the veggies and toss to coat. Then sprinkle on a teaspoon (5 g) of the Indian Seasoning Blend and toss again to evenly distribute the spices.

Lay the veggies on a parchment-lined baking sheet in a single layer, leaving an inch or so (about 2 cm) between the veggies so they are able to roast. If the veggies crowd, they will bake instead.

Roast for 20 to 25 minutes, turning the veggies over at 15 minutes. Once they're removed from the oven, sprinkle with a pinch of coarse sea salt and allow to cool on a rack or laid out in a single layer. Piling these up while hot may make them mushy. Let them cool down a bit before mounding up.

These are great dipped in a Paleo mayo or ketchup, but a sauce is not necessary. They make a great side dish to simple grilled or roasted chicken for an easy weeknight dinner. It'll only taste fancy.

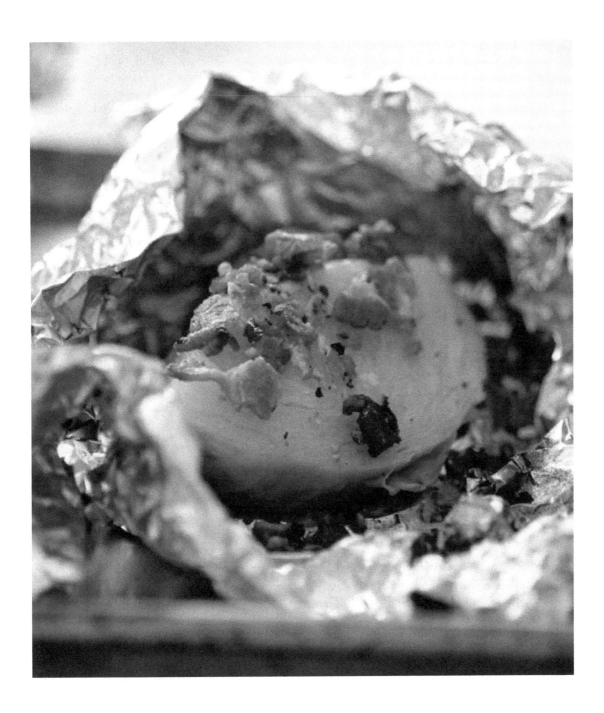

CABBAGE PACKAGES

A humble head of cabbage is transformed into something truly side-dish worthy thanks to the magic of the aluminum foil packet and a few favorite ingredients. Set aside some leftover bacon for this one; your summer barbecues have been missing these cabbage packages.

Serves 4 to 8

1 head organic cabbage

2 cloves garlic

1 lemon

4 or 5 slices cooked bacon

Sea salt and black pepper, to taste

Fresh chopped Italian flat-leaf parsley, to garnish

Preheat the oven to 400°F (204°C).

Quarter the head of cabbage into wedges and trim off most of the inedible core.

Mince the garlic and divide into four portions, but leave them on the cutting board. Roll the lemon to get the juices flowing and cut it in half. Chop the cooked bacon slices and set aside— anywhere between a third cup to a half cup (75 g to 115 g) is the right amount.

Build the packages by laying down a sheet of foil large enough to comfortably wrap around the size of cabbage wedge you have in front of you. Place a cabbage wedge on the foil and squeeze half the juice from the lemon half over the cabbage on the cut sides, focusing in on the tight layers so the juice really gets into it.

Top the wedge with a quarter of the minced garlic, some salt and pepper to taste, plus a couple tablespoons (32 g) of bacon bits.

Seal the package by bringing the long sides together and folding together several times until it reaches the top of the cabbage. Then roll each end up in the same fashion to seal the package completely. Repeat this process for all four wedges.

Bake for 25 minutes. It's a good idea to keep the packages sealed until meal time. The flavors will continue to develop and the cabbage will soften. When the time comes to serve, top the wedges with the package contents plus some fresh chopped Italian flat-leaf parsley.

To really send this over the moon, I recommend serving with Homemade Mayonnaise from here on the side for dipping.

HARD CIDER SPROUTS

This recipe is a spin-off of Hard Cider Braised Brats, which you can find on here. Brussels sprouts and hard apple cider are a perfect flavor combination; I just can't get enough of this recipe. Five main ingredients and about 20 minutes, and you've a distinct side dish that will keep people guessing!

Serves 2 to 4

---

1 tbsp (15 g) lard or bacon drippings

1 lb (454 g) Brussels sprouts, trimmed and halved

¼ cup (40 g) white or yellow onion, diced

1 bay leaf

Salt and black pepper, to taste

1 cup (273 mL) hard apple cider, gluten-free, with no sugar added

Heat a large skillet over medium-high heat and melt the lard or bacon drippings.

Drop in the sprouts, onion and the whole bay leaf. Season with salt and black pepper to your preference. Pan roast (meaning keep the temperature at medium-high and don't move the veggies around as often as in sautéing) until the sprouts take on some color and the onion softens and becomes translucent—about 8 to 10 minutes. You'll notice that the bottom of the pan has started to collect brown bits as the fat is absorbed into the veggies and they caramelize. This is exactly what we want to see.

Deglaze with the hard apple cider to lift all those brown bits from the pan. Cook and stir until the bits are absorbed into the cider and the cider reduces by at least half, about 5 to 10 minutes. The goal is to create a light glaze as opposed to a soupy sauce for the sprouts.

Remove and discard the bay leaf. Serve the sprouts hot.

SUMMER STRAWBERRY SALAD WITH CHOCOLATE BALSAMIC VINAIGRETTE

I was having lunch with a couple of friends at this great little sandwich and salad shop when I first came across something that changed my world forever—chocolate balsamic vinaigrette. Here is the simplified version of what I ate at that unforgettable lunch. Enjoy it on a warm summer's day when strawberries and fresh spinach are at their best.

Serves 4

FOR THE SALAD

5 cups (190 g) organic baby spinach

1 cup (200 g) sliced organic strawberries

1 tsp (4 g) chia seeds, to garnish (optional)

FOR THE VINAIGRETTE

1 tsp (5 g) raw cacao

1 tbsp (15 mL) avocado oil

3 tbsp (45 mL) good-quality balsamic vinegar

In a large mixing bowl, toss the spinach and sliced strawberries together.

In a separate bowl, build the vinaigrette. First combine the raw cacao and avocado oil with a whisk until smooth. Raw cacao can be quite fine, so take care that all of the lumps are worked out. Next stream in the balsamic vinegar, whisking as it is streamed in to thoroughly combine, or emulsify, with the avocado oil. That's it.

Drizzle the chocolate balsamic vinaigrette over the spinach and strawberries, tossing gently to evenly coat the salad in the dressing. Sprinkle with chia seeds, if using, and serve right away.

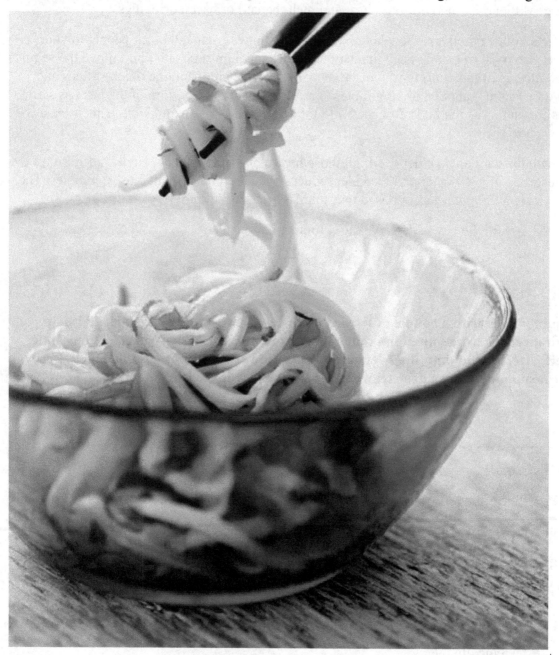

ZOODLES WITH CHILIES AND VINEGAR

You'll need to have a spiral cutter or julienne peeler in order to cut whole zucchini into noodle-like shapes, which we in Paleo affectionately refer to as "zoodles." Zoodles are commonly par-cooked and used as a pasta substitute, but this recipe serves them raw and flavored boldly with Asian-inspired ingredients.

Serves 4 to 6

---

2 (6 inch [15 cm]) organic zucchini

2 red chili peppers

¼ cup (60 mL) coconut vinegar or rice wine vinegar

½ cup (25 g) thinly sliced green onions (sliced on the bias)

Trim the ends from the zucchini and cut into "noodles," ideally using a spiral cutting tool or a julienne peeler. Place in a large mixing bowl.

Remove the stems from the red chilies, slice open lengthwise and remove the seeds and ribs. I like to use a pair of latex-free gloves when working with peppers since the oils are easily absorbed into skin and can cause burning. If you don't have gloves, just be sure to thoroughly wash your hands after dicing the peppers and do not touch your eyes, nose or face! Once the ribs are removed, finely dice the chilies.

Pour the vinegar into a medium mixing bowl. Add the red chilies and green onions. Mix together and then pour over the zucchini. Toss to evenly distribute.

Serve cold or at room temperature. If the salad rests at all prior to serving, be sure to give it a fresh toss before dishing up. The vinegar will pool at the bottom as it sits.

CHILI AND CACAO ROASTED CAULIFLOWER

Quite possibly my new favorite way to eat cauliflower, this recipe combines some unlikely ingredients. Spicy, earthy ancho chili powder partnered with savory raw cacao complements roasted cauliflower in a way that you have to try for yourself to believe! I buy my raw cacao in the bulk section of my local health food store and use spoonfuls of it here and there to enhance recipes or green smoothies. Using large quantities of cacao in treats can get expensive, but small amounts in special recipes stretches the purchase.

Serves 4

---

1 head organic cauliflower

½ tsp ancho chili powder

½ tsp raw cacao

½ tsp kosher salt

1 tbsp (15 g) coconut oil

Preheat the grill to 450°F (232°C).

To prepare the cauliflower, remove the leaves and core and cut into florets. The florets should be on the large size, quite comparable to the floret that forms naturally within the head. Place the florets in a medium bowl.

In a small bowl, mix together the ancho chili powder, raw cacao and kosher salt. Melt the coconut oil. Add the oil to the florets and toss. Then add the chili powder mixture and toss again.

Transfer to a grill basket and roast for 20 to 25 minutes, or until the cauliflower is al dente and has caramelized a bit. Serve warm.

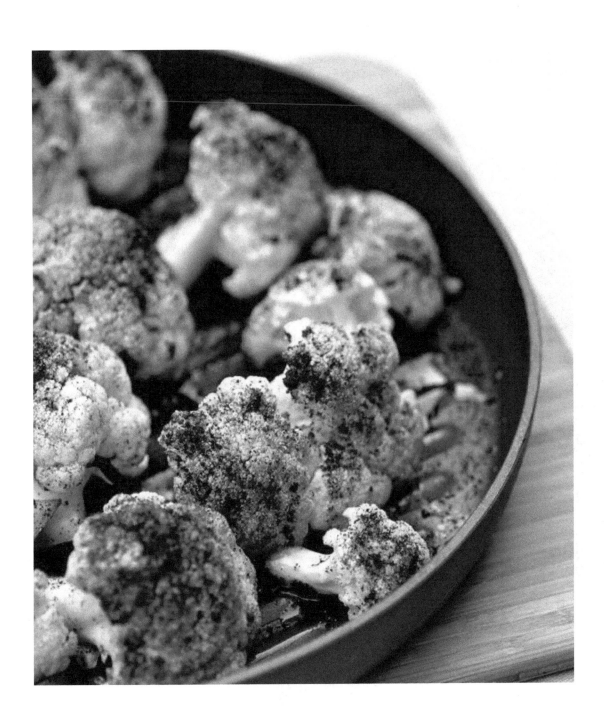

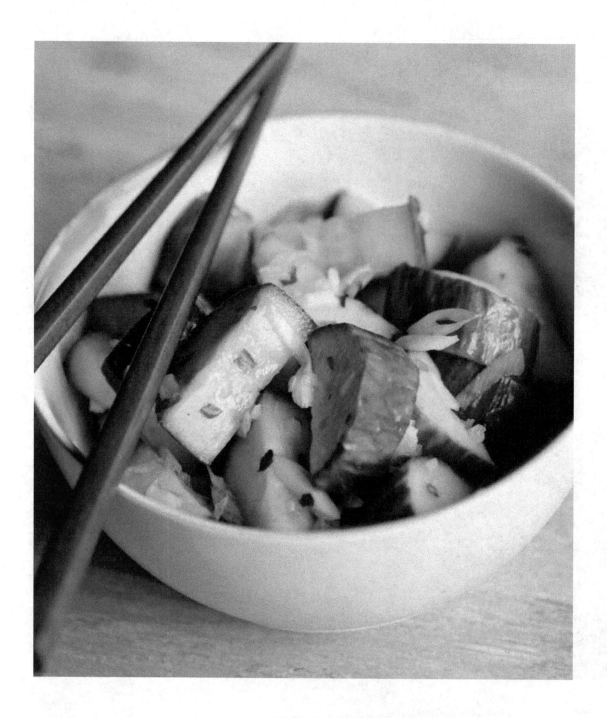

CHEATER CUCUMBER KIM CHEE

I enjoy traditional kim chee, but my favorite version is made with seedless cucumber and is eaten fresh as opposed to fermented. Because many of my readers say they tend to avoid recipes that they feel are overly complicated or use ingredients that are not easy to find, I've modified one of my favorite kim chee recipes to use readily available ingredients with minimal steps to prepare. Instead of using fine Korean red-pepper flakes, grab a bottle of regular crushed red-pepper flakes and enjoy this cheater version.

Serves 2 to 4

1 English cucumber

2 tbsp (30 g) kosher salt

2 cups (474 mL) cold water

2 cloves garlic

1 tsp (5 g) crushed red-pepper flakes

1 tbsp (5 g) thinly sliced green onions

Start by preparing the English cucumber. These are the seedless kind that generally come individually wrapped and do not require peeling. Remove the wrapper, wash the cucumber skin, trim away the ends and cut the cucumber in half lengthwise. Then cut each half into half-inch (1.25-cm) slices, or half-moon shapes.

Put the cucumber in a bowl and add the kosher salt and cold water. Mix it up to help dissolve the salt a bit, then soak for about 10 minutes. Drain the salted water and rinse the cucumber in cold water. Don't worry about drying the cucumber off; a little bit of residual water isn't going to hurt.

Mince the garlic cloves very well, to the point of creating a paste. To help break it down, use the flat side of the knife. Lay the flat of the knife over the cloves with the sharp edge of the blade angled down toward the cutting board so you don't cut yourself. With a swift hand, give the flat side a slam to further crush the garlic underneath. Then, while applying pressure to the knife, slide it across the garlic to smear it into a paste. Repeat this a couple of times to thoroughly break down the garlic.

In a small bowl, combine the garlic with the crushed red-pepper flakes and green onions. Then add the mixture to the cucumber slices and toss to combine. Notice how the residual water from the earlier rinse helps to move the garlic and pepper flakes over the cucumber and create a sauce of sorts.

Serve the fresh kim chee right away. It can also be held in an airtight container in the refrigerator for a few days, but it will begin to break down and ferment within a day, resulting in a texture that may not be ideal. I find a fresh, crisp cucumber is better than a softened, fermented one for this recipe—though it is still fine to eat.

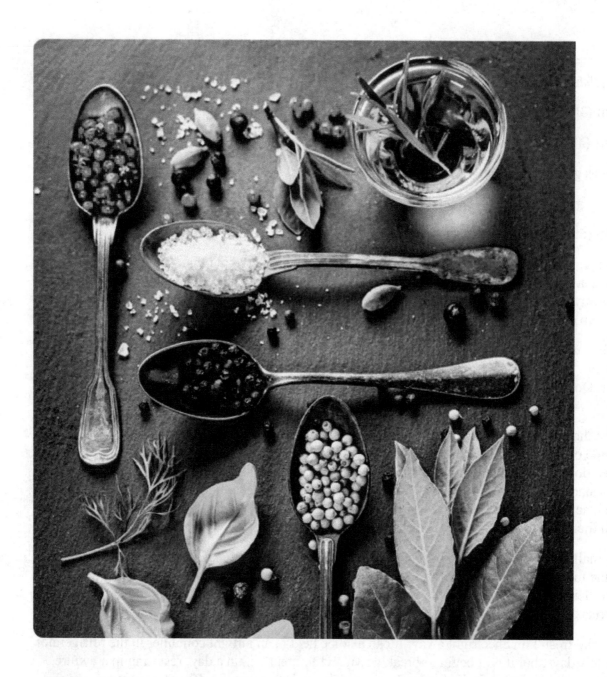

When it comes to preparing delicious and frugal Paleo meals, there are a few timeless tricks of the trade. I'm convinced that anyone can stay the course with the following methods:

• Make friends with your spice rack: Use spice regularly and with intention.

• Think Next-Meal Potential: How many meals can you get out of one basic recipe?

• Weekly staples: Identify the basics you eat regularly and make them in advance.

SPICE THINGS UP

One of the keys to making delicious, affordable meals that you see used throughout this book is spice. I like to use different, but accessible, spices and herbs with creativity and intention. Instead of a pinch of this and a dash of that, enhance a basic food item, like mushrooms for example, with bold and dominant flavors. The garlic and red-pepper flakes in Mushroom Diavolo (here) create an explosion of flavor in your mouth. It tastes anything but plain, and yet the whole recipe is comprised of only four main ingredients. Partner those mushrooms with a grilled steak, preferably one that you've thawed from your annual quarter-cow purchase, and you've just created a memorable, simple and affordable meal that anyone can enjoy—Paleo or not!

It was in this spirit that I developed the fifteen Salt-Free, 5-Ingredients-or-Less Seasoning Blends. No matter which direction you want to take a boring vegetable or a plain piece of protein, these seasoning blends have you covered. They use five or fewer different seasonings to create various profiles, and all of the seasonings can be found in the spice section of your regular grocery store.

THINK NEXT-MEAL POTENTIAL

Constantly be mindful of next-meal potential. This keeps me focused on choosing recipes that I know are either cost-efficient enough on their own for a single meal or have enough value in terms of extending beyond the primary recipe, which justifies spending more in most cases.

Make relatively flexible recipes like Pork Tacos 101 (here) and roll the leftovers forward into breakfast the next day with Santa Fe Skillet (here). And if you still have leftovers from the pork, enjoy it reheated with a baked sweet potato and Easy Avocado Lime Salad (here) for lunch. Planning meals and shopping for ingredients that pair well with each other in varied combinations for breakfast, lunch and dinner will maximize your grocery purchases every time no matter what great eats you're serving up!

WEEKLY STAPLES

Weekly staples look different for every family. My family are big snackers; it seems that the moment someone walks into the house, the first thing they want is something to munch on. So for us our weekly staples are Charps (here), Plantain Chips (here) with Spinach Guacamole Salsa (here), Scotch Eggs (here) or leftover meatballs that can be warmed up and served with a few slices of avocado and hot sauce. Since Paleo is not a fast-food game, preparing go-to favorites ahead of time is key for us.

Beyond snacks, there are several foods that we have come to rely on for weekly meal preparation. Bone broth, poached chicken and homemade mayonnaise have become three critical items in my house. Since I can anticipate that we will need to have these items on hand for whipping up easy chicken lettuce wraps, egg or tuna salads, and for thinning soups and sauces, I make it a habit of prepping those items in advance every week. It saves me money and time having the foods I know we will need on hand and waiting for us—rather than us waiting for them. We enjoy our meals knowing that the most nutrient-rich ingredients available are on our plates and that we didn't pay out the nose for any of it. Okay, so maybe I'm the one who enjoys that part. The others are just hungry and are too busy gobbling up their yummy meals….

Here are 15 ways to spice up those boring meals as well as recipes for the six staples of the Popular Paleo Household.

15 SALT-FREE, 5-INGREDIENTS-OR-LESS SEASONING BLENDS

To get right to the point, I don't like bland food. I have found that the easiest way to make Paleo meals taste great is to not skimp on spice. But here's the thing—it doesn't have to be expensive or rare to be flavorful and distinctive. To illustrate to you how much you can do with common foods and spices, I've created a list of 15 seasoning blends that are salt free and each use only five ingredients or fewer. You may have to hit up the grocery store for one or two of these items, but in general, these are all common household seasonings.

So why salt free?

First of all, we have different palates. Some prefer more salt, some prefer less. Some prefer more prominent, bold-tasting salts like table or kosher, and others appreciate the more subtle or rich-tasting flavors that come from sea salts. But it's not always a personal preference. Recipes vary and taking this tact of a salt-free seasoning blend lets the overall recipe dictate the salt quantity required.

Another reason for not including salt in these blends is because it comes in various types and grains. From standard table salt to kosher and others with higher mineral content like Celtic and Himalayan varieties, the kind of salt chosen brings with it a spectrum of flavors and intensity. Depending on the dish, one variety may make more sense over another. For example, table salt is ideal for fermenting kim chee. However, Celtic sea salt is a perfect finisher for chocolate truffles. Taste and texture matter.

In terms of grain size, I like to use coarse-grain sea salt for finishing dishes, whereas finer grain like kosher salt is better in recipes that call for ground meat. Obviously, the finer the grain the more effectively and evenly the dish will be salted, achieving balanced flavor. In some cases, the recipe is actually improved with isolated, pronounced grains of salt such as to finish roasted vegetables fresh from the oven or sprinkled over a simple hard-cooked egg.

Lastly, this method is perfect for roasting vegetables or making chips. Since salt draws out moisture, chips won't crisp if the seasoning blend contains salt. Pick a blend from this list, season your desired vegetable prior to cooking and then season with salt once it is fresh from the oven.

HOUSE SEASONING BLEND

Yield: Approximately 1 tbsp (15 g)

1 tsp (3 g) garlic

1 tsp (3 g) onion powder

¼ tsp ground cayenne pepper

½ tsp ground black pepper

In a small bowl, combine all ingredients and mix well.

Find this seasoning blend in: Eggplant Sliders (here), Tuesday Night Chicken (here), Crispy Chicken with Lemon and Capers (here), Summer Prawn Salad (here) and Eggplant Tomato Skillet (here).

TACO SEASONING BLEND

Yield: Approximately 1 tbsp (15 g)

½ tsp ground cumin

½ tsp ground coriander

½ tsp onion powder

1 tsp (3 g) garlic powder

½ tsp chili powder

In a small bowl, combine all ingredients and mix well.

Find this seasoning blend in: Ultimate Taco Meat (here), Tequila Carnitas (here), Pork Tacos 101 (here), Slow Cooker Taco Soup (here) and Tex-Mex Casserole (here).

FAJITA SEASONING BLEND

Yield: Approximately 1 tbsp (15 g)

¼ tsp chipotle chili powder

1 tsp (4 g) ground coriander

¼ tsp ground black pepper

1 tsp (4 g) dried oregano

¼ tsp ground cayenne pepper

In a small bowl, combine all ingredients and mix well.

Find this seasoning blend in: Barbacoa (here), Zesty Turkey Meatballs (here) and Braised Chicken Fajitas (here).

CLASSIC RANCH SEASONING

Yield: Approximately 1 tbsp (15 g)

---

1 tsp (4 g) dried dillweed

1 tsp (4 g) dried parsley

½ tsp garlic powder

½ tsp onion powder

¼ tsp ground black pepper

In a small bowl, combine all ingredients and mix well.

Find this seasoning blend in: Bacon-Ranch Chicken (here) and Paleo Hotdish (here).

BBQ SEASONING BLEND

Yield: Approximately 1 tbsp (15 g)

---

1 tsp (4 g) chili powder

1 tsp (4 g) onion powder

½ tsp smoked paprika

½ tsp ground black pepper

¼ tsp ground mustard

In a small bowl, combine all ingredients and mix well.

Find this seasoning blend in: Oven BBQ Pork Chops (here).

ITALIAN SEASONING BLEND

Yield: Approximately 1 tbsp (15 g)

---

1 tsp (4 g) dried basil

1 tsp (4 g) dried oregano

½ tsp dried marjoram

½ tsp dried thyme

¼ tsp crushed red-pepper flakes

In a small bowl, combine all ingredients and mix well.

Find this seasoning blend in: Mushroom Skillet Lasagna (here), Tuesday Night Chicken (here), Poor Man's Braciole (here) and Chunky Garden Chicken Cacciatore (here).

CREOLE SEASONING BLEND

Yield: Approximately 1 tbsp (15 g)

½ tsp smoked paprika

1 tsp (3 g) garlic powder

½ tsp dried thyme

½ tsp dried oregano

¼ tsp ground black pepper

In a small bowl, combine all ingredients and mix well.

Find this seasoning blend in: Creole-Style Marrow (here) and Creole Baked Cod (here).

BLACKENING SEASONING BLEND

Yield: Approximately 1 tbsp (15 g)

½ tsp ground black pepper

½ tsp ground white pepper

¼ tsp ground cayenne pepper

1 tsp (3 g) garlic powder

1 tsp (3 g) onion powder

In a small bowl, combine all ingredients and mix well.

Find this seasoning blend in: Oven-Blackened Pulled Pork (here) and Triple-Pepper Lemon Chicken (here).

JERK SEASONING BLEND

Yield: Approximately 1 tbsp (15 g)

---

1 tsp (3 g) Jamaican allspice

1 tsp (3 g) onion powder

½ tsp dried thyme

¼ tsp ground cayenne pepper

¼ tsp ground black pepper

In a small bowl, combine all ingredients and mix well.

Find this seasoning blend in: Oven-Roasted Jerk Chicken (here).

ASIAN SEASONING BLEND

Yield: Approximately 1 tbsp (15 g)

½ tsp Chinese five-spice

1 tsp (4 g) toasted sesame seeds

½ tsp garlic powder

¼ tsp ground coriander

In a small bowl, combine all ingredients and mix well.

INDIAN SEASONING BLEND

Yield: Approximately 1 tbsp (15 g)

¾ tsp ground cumin

¾ tsp ground coriander

¾ tsp garlic powder

½ tsp ground ginger

¼ tsp ground cinnamon

In a small bowl, combine all ingredients and mix well.

Find this seasoning blend in: Ginger Peach Pulled Pork (here), Bombay Parsnip and Carrot Fries (here) and Punjabi Cabbage (here).

BREAKFAST SEASONING BLEND

Yield: Approximately 1 tsp (5 g)

½ tsp ground cinnamon

⅛ tsp ground nutmeg

⅛ tsp ground cloves

In a small bowl, combine all ingredients and mix well.

Find this seasoning blend in: Apple Butternut Hash (here).

AUTUMN SEASONING BLEND

Yield: Approximately 1 tbsp (15 g)

½ tsp dried sage

1 tsp (3 g) dried thyme

½ tsp fennel seeds

½ tsp onion powder

¼ tsp ground white pepper

In a small bowl, combine all ingredients and mix well.

Find this seasoning blend in: Roasted Carrot Soup (here).

FRENCH COUNTRYSIDE SEASONING BLEND

Yield: Approximately 1 tbsp (15 g)

½ tsp dried rosemary

½ tsp dried marjoram

½ tsp dried thyme

½ tsp onion powder

¼ tsp fennel seeds

In a small bowl, combine all ingredients and mix well.

Find this seasoning blend in: Roasted French Countryside Chicken (here).

ADOBO SEASONING BLEND

Yield: Approximately 1 tbsp (15 g)

---

1 tsp (3 g) dried oregano

½ tsp ground cumin

½ tsp ancho chili powder

½ tsp garlic powder

½ tsp onion powder

In a small bowl, combine all ingredients and mix well.

Find this seasoning blend in: Chicken and Chorizo Stew (here).

PLANTAIN CHIPS

Most commonly used as a substitute for tortilla chips, plantain chips are a good source of grain-free carbohydrates and are an ideal vessel for getting more nutrient-dense and metabolically supportive coconut oil into your diet. I find that I make a batch or two a week for my own snacks as well as for my kids; they love them! I also use them to make Chilaquiles on here. And a bonus? They are cheap! No need to buy them by the bunch the way we buy bananas; one or two plantains go a long way.

Serves 2

---

1 green (unripe) plantain, peeled

1 tbsp (15 g) Paleo-friendly preferred fat, melted (I like coconut oil or lard)

Pinch of sea salt

Preheat the oven to 350°F (177°C).

Use a mandoline to cut the plantain into ⅛-inch (3-mm) slices. If you don't have a mandoline, grab your favorite knife and get to work. As long as the slices are uniformly sliced as thin as you can get them, they will turn out.

In a medium bowl, toss the plantain slices with your melted fat of choice. For plantain chips, I prefer to use coconut oil, but freshly rendered lard from pastured pigs is quite tasty as well.

Bake on a baking sheet lined with parchment or a silicone mat for 20 to 25 minutes. Plantains require babysitting during those last few minutes thanks to their natural sugars. They can go from perfect to burnt in seconds.

When the chips are golden brown and crisp, remove from the oven, transfer to a bowl and toss in a pinch of sea salt as quickly as possible. The salt sticks better if it's hitting hot chips versus cool ones.

HOMEMADE MAYONNAISE

Once you get the feel for making mayonnaise at home, I'm willing to bet you will be hard-pressed to buy it from the grocery store ever again. The amount of quality flavor (and quality fat) that homemade provides is unparalleled in the processed food world. This weekly staple partners well with canned tuna, hard-cooked eggs or shredded poached chicken for quick cold salads, giving you a familiar lunch or snack in minutes. I also find it handy for mixing up tasty dipping sauces. Combine a bit of mayo with any of the 15 Salt-Free, Five-Ingredient-or-Less Seasonings Blends and you've got a custom dipping sauce for Sweet Potato Tater Tots (here), Creole Baked Cod (here) or Cabbage Packages (here).

Keeping things as simple as possible, these are the best and least expensive ingredients required to whip up some fresh mayonnaise in your own kitchen. Intimidated? Don't be. It's so much easier than you might think. Mayo is a basic emulsion, which means you're bringing together ingredients which on their own would not combine. Simply stirring oil with egg yolks would yield … oil on top of some mixed-up egg yolk. However, a slow drizzling of oil while vigorously whisking eggs produces a thick and creamy emulsion. The trick? Room temperature ingredients are the key to making the mayo magic happen. Let me show you….

Yield: 1 ½ cups (330 g)

---

2 egg yolks, at room temperature

1 tsp (3 g) ground mustard

1 tbsp (15 mL) apple cider vinegar

1 tbsp (15 mL) water

1 cup (237 mL) avocado oil (or a light-tasting olive oil, not extra virgin)

½ tsp kosher salt

Place the egg yolks, ground mustard, vinegar and water in your mixing vessel. I prefer to use a food processor or high-speed blender, though many people have success with an immersion blender. It's your choice. Even whisking by hand works, if you're up for a workout.

Turn the food processor on and slowly (and I mean s-l-o-w-l-y) pour in the oil. Drizzling the oil allows it to emulsify with the egg, making the mayo magic happen. It should take a few minutes to get all the way through the whole cup if you're doing it right.

When the emulsion is complete, turn off the processor. Scrape down the sides and under the blade—anywhere that you see unmixed ingredients. Add in the kosher salt. Pulse the processor a couple of times to incorporate, and that's it! You've made mayonnaise!

Transfer to an airtight container and store in the refrigerator. Because there are no preservatives in your homemade mayo, it will have a shelf life. The mayo is fresh as long as the egg is, so be sure to note the expiration date of your eggs and transfer that date over.

9 781915 032270